THE PRENATAL BOMBSHELL

THE PRENATAL BOMBSHELL

Help and Hope When Continuing or Ending a Precious Pregnancy after an Abnormal Diagnosis

Stephanie Azri and Sherokee Ilse

ROWMAN & LITTLEFIELD
Lanham • Boulder • New York • London

Published by Rowman & Littlefield
A wholly owned subsidiary of The Rowman & Littlefield Publishing Group,
Inc.
4501 Forbes Boulevard, Suite 200, Lanham, Maryland 20706
www.rowman.com

Unit A, Whitacre Mews, 26-34 Stannary Street, London SE11 4AB

British Library Cataloguing in Publication Information Available

Library of Congress Cataloging-in-Publication Data

Azri, Stephanie, 1977- , author.
The prenatal bombshell : help and hope when continuing or ending a precious pregnancy after an
abnormal diagnosis / Stephanie Azri and Sherokee Ilse.
p. ; cm.
Includes bibliographical references.
ISBN 978-1-4422-3942-5 (cloth : alk. paper) -- ISBN 978-1-4422-3943-2 (electronic)
I. Ilse, Sherokee, author. II. Title.
[DNLM: 1. Decision Making--Personal Narratives. 2. Prenatal Diagnosis--psychology--Personal
Narratives. 3. Abortion, Induced--Personal Narratives. 4. Bereavement--Personal Narratives. 5.
Patient Education as Topic--Personal Narratives. WQ 209]
RG628
618.3'2075--dc23
2014040890

∞™ The paper used in this publication meets the minimum requirements of
American National Standard for Information Sciences Permanence of Paper
for Printed Library Materials, ANSI/NISO Z39.48-1992.

Printed in the United States of America

CONTENTS

FOREWORD

Kiley Hanish

We've all been told that pregnancy is a time of joy, hope, and anticipation. It's a time to pick colors, paint rooms, and ready ourselves for the parenting adventure of a lifetime.

We begin planning for the future the moment we discover we are expecting. We change our eating habits—swapping folic acid for Fumé Blanc—stretching our mortgage to move into a neighborhood with better schools, listing baby names that—at the time—we think will make or break our little bambino's (or bambina's) future.

In all of our decisions, no matter how big or small, the newest member of the family—the one we can't wait to meet—is always front and center. Unfortunately, that's all the joy some couples will ever experience.

Too soon, many discover their beloved children will not survive or will have serious medical problems that will result in fetal death or an impaired life. These couples have to make the impossible and most heartbreaking decision of all—whether to continue or end the pregnancy.

Neither is an easy decision, nor is there a right one that fits everyone.

Understandably, parents in these situations often experience isolation, guilt, shame, grief, depression, and anxiety. No matter what decision they make, they need support to help them make it through the darkest days and nights when they don't think they can go on another minute. They need to know that there is hope, they need to see a glimpse of light, and they need to see that there is joy and meaning in life after this.

When my husband and I made the film *Return to Zero* about the loss of our son, Norbert, at the end of our first pregnancy, we did so in order to open up a discussion about stillbirth and neonatal loss. We hope that we have made a small dent in the universe and allowed those who suffer in silence to know that they are not alone. That there are others out there who share in their pain, their experience, and are there to help.

In *The Prenatal Bombshell: Help and Hope When Continuing or Ending a Precious Pregnancy after an Abnormal Diagnosis*, Sherokee and Stephanie have done the same for another group of parents who struggle and suffer in silence. They draw from their own experiences of the deaths of their children to offer specific support about how to live through the aftermath of making the most harrowing and difficult decision any parent could possibly make.

The book offers unbiased, nonjudgmental strategies for finding your way on this most challenging path, and they give their "love and hope to instill the belief that *you can make it*. You can put your world back together, despite the devastation from the bombshell that was suddenly dropped on your happy, hopeful life."

That is why this book is a gift to so many.

Many parents' touching stories are beautifully woven into the text to show you that you are not alone. That you are a part of a larger community that has been through the same. They share their stories so that you can know they are profoundly changed in amazing and beautiful ways by their babies' lives, no matter how brief. Sometimes it takes a long time to see these changes, "but with an open attitude and heart, you can feel it and find it when you are ready. Embrace those gifts and recognize the light, which shines even in the darkness."

Whether you have chosen to continue or have ended your pregnancy, they offer tips, strategies, and advice to help you cope with your own emotions; deal with your friends, family, and community; communicate with your spouse or partner; and care for your living children in the aftermath.

You will be offered ideas for bonding and making memories both with your baby who is in the womb, as well as when the child is born still or alive. These are so very important. Despite the fact that your baby may die, he or she is still your baby. Your child did live inside of you, and the time you have with him or her is sacred.

Life "down the road" is also discussed in detail. How do you go back to work? Find a new focus? What are normal grief reactions? How does one heal? They talk about how to cope with subsequent pregnancies and births. There is a future, but seeing it from where you stand now can be so very difficult.

I wish I had some of the information in this book when I learned that my son Norbert died. I wish I wasn't so afraid and could have cherished our very special time together. I do know that my Norbert's life has been a gift and transformed me as a person, and I am grateful for his life in so many ways now that I never knew then.

This book will come to be regarded as a lifesaving guide for families who are enduring these types of situations. I sincerely hope you find something in these pages as I have, and I believe that you will.

With love,
Kiley

Kiley Krekorian Hanish, OTD, OTR/L,
Co-creator, *Return to Zero* (www.returntozerothemovie.com),
the first film that featured stillbirth as a central theme

PREFACE

The deeper that sorrow carves into your being, the more joy you can contain. Is not the cup that holds your wine the very cup that was burned in the potter's oven? —Kahlil Gibran

I am humbled to witness how the most traumatic loss of my life also turned into the most life-changing event for me as a mother, as a woman, and as a professional. Being told at twenty weeks in 2002 that my baby would die changed me forever. The shock, the shattering of my innocence, and the heartbreaking pregnancy options I was given affected me a great deal to say the least. Watching little Talina be born at home and die a couple of hours later gave me a reason to look at my life with new lenses. I suppose tragedy has a way of making people reconsider their lives, choices, and priorities. And Talina did exactly that for me. Her death broke me, and I was reborn a better person. Through this process, though, there were times when I thought I would not survive and begged for just a little relief from my grief. After a while, I slowly learned to put one foot in front of the other, and I learned that I could honor Talina's short life in so many beautiful ways.

My research, my career, my books, and PDS Australia (a prenatal diagnosis support group found at www.PDSAustralia.org) is her legacy. Who I am as a mother and as a person today is her gift to me. I want to share this gift with you. I want to tell you that you will survive this journey, that you are not alone, and that your baby, no matter your decision about your pregnancy, will be with you forever. Feel free to contact me through my Facebook page (Stephanie Azri Author). If by reading this book you feel a little bit of hope, then we'll have accomplished our humble wish.

—Stephanie Azri

Being a bereaved mother has changed me deeply through the years. There were surely many days, months, and even times during the passing years when I cried lots, reviewed our story, and wallowed in the pain and sadness of it all. Thankfully, in time I came to realize that there is more to our babies' short lives than that. I changed and grew, coming to understand that because of our abiding love for our babies, great joys and a new perspective on life have come. I feel honored to be Marama, Brennan, and Bryna's mother. Their short lives contributed to the future we enjoy with our sons Kellan and Trevor. I now truly believe that our sons would not be here but for their siblings who came before, and I cannot imagine our lives without them. I have parented differently—more intentionally present and outwardly expressing my love. Gratefulness flows through my heart daily, despite life's turmoil and challenges.

This book is a gift from my heart to yours. I pray that my experience and the insights from others will touch you and teach you. That you will feel empowered to be your child's parent and to be present and intentional about how you live through this loss and go forward, to still "love and love again."

—Sherokee Ilse

Life is a journey with many twists and turns. No one knows what is ahead, only what is behind. Embrace each precious day: the sun and the rain, the wind and the storm, and the chaos and calm at the end of the day. We are at one with each other and our loved ones, no matter where they reside. Peace is waiting to be reached and held.

As you travel forth, our wish for you is to . . .

Know deep in your heart that you are not alone and not the only one who has traveled this road. Keep looking for your sisters and brothers within this community of parents who embrace the everlasting love of their children.

Feel supported and understood. You can find people, including many compassionate care providers, parents, groups, websites, social media groups, books, and videos that can affirm feelings of being supported and understood. People who can finish your sentences for you. People who do not judge you but love you though you have never met. People who care for you in your darkest hours. Feel that love.

Share your children with others. Say their names out loud. Proudly. Boldly. Lovingly. They have graced this earth and wrapped themselves around the hearts of many, especially you and their families.

Honor them in meaningful ways. By keeping their memories alive in your family and at special family gatherings. As you reach out to others in their name. When you create, write, make music, build, teach, touch, give to others, and love.

Love every minute you had with them. In time, you can release the pain and heartache. It is and always has been about *love*, and hope, and family, and relationships. Feel that love. Grow that love. Give that love to each other and to yourself.

ACKNOWLEDGMENTS

We are grateful for all who provided support and advice to us while writing this book. As professionals and experts in this field, we are strong believers that we do not—and should not—work in isolation for this great purpose. When we collaborate, richness follows. We feel blessed for the input, advice, and concern about our project that many bereaved parents and professionals have provided to us, creating a much better book. We are grateful to the following people in no particular order:

Thank you to our families who sacrificed and shared us with our computers during the past two years: our husbands Sid Azri and David Ilse; our living children Julianna, Killian, Phoenix, Jett, and Noah Azri and Kellan and Trevor Ilse (and their partners). And of course, we both appreciate the gifts given to us by our children who died too soon, Talina Azri and Brennan William, Marama, and Bryna Ilse.

A special thanks to our colleagues and readers who shared thoughtful contributions, which help make this book real, raw, and more readable: Tracy Ahrens, Stephanie and Andy Barbieri, Angie and Cecil Bellephant, Julie Bryant, Vicki Culling, Lori Spray-Esteve, Lisa Foster, Amy Kuelbebeck, Nathalie Himmelrich, Ivy Margulies, Lori Martini, Jennifer Ross, Sue Steen, Bina Vora Taibi, Danielle Townsend, Toni-Marie Vlearbone, and others not mentioned. Many of these are parents whose inspiration comes from their babies who died too soon.

Thank you Kiley Hanish for your willingness to open this special book with your words of wisdom and love. By sharing your story in

Return to Zero, the first full-length drama with stillbirth as its subject, your family, including your stillborn son Norbert, has touched the hearts of millions of people throughout the world. And your kind and insightful foreword is an invitation for readers to feel our love, support, and guidance during a most tragic and overwhelming time in their lives.

Thank you Rowman & Littlefield for publishing this very important book. Thank you to our editor, Suzanne Staszak-Silva, who was much more than an editor. She showed passion, care, and dedication, wanting only the best for families with a poor prenatal diagnosis.

And, most importantly, to all the families who provided their testimonies, thank you from the bottom of our hearts. We know how difficult it can be to share those experiences. Yet they were willing to do so in hopes that others in similar situations might feel their love and learn about what is to come in their journey after making a life-altering decision. Their beautiful quotes and stories bring to life messages of love and hope.

We dedicate this book to their babies' memories and to all those beloved babies who may die or have serious life challenges in the years ahead. While they are yet to be born, we already know the depth of their parents' love. We sincerely hope that through this collaborative work, their parents' burdens will be lightened.

INTRODUCTION

Setting the Stage

IF YOU ARE A PROFESSIONAL

Although this book is written primarily for parents, it is also written for professionals. Genetic counselors, perinatal clinic staff, perinatologists, perinatal hospice staff, and all who work with these families: you are key professionals during a fatal or life-altering diagnosis and beyond. Many parents share how grateful they are to you; we want you to know that your work and gifts make a huge difference! Some parents report that they felt they weren't given enough of a sense of reality about their options. They wonder if there had been such guidance, would they have made a different choice or been more prepared for the decision they made. It is our hope that when you read this book, you will be reminded of the lifelong impact and importance of your words, guidance, and the many existing resources to assist families at the time of diagnosis and as they go forward.

When you help parents in a neutral fashion, it is most beneficial that you help them be fully informed and that you understand the profound consequences of either decision, of what they may encounter on either path. Will you show that you have hope that they can survive the journey and get support in either case? The more you learn about perinatal hospice, for example, the more comfortable you might be, knowing that it is a viable option and that there is much support for continuing a pregnancy. We mention that because parents have told us that although both options were presented, too often, continuing the pregnancy was not a choice offered wholeheartedly. They wonder if it might be because the professionals caring for them were unfamiliar with perinatal hospice and all the available information that is out there (including such books as this and other resources about continuing a pregnancy). And they wonder if it might be due to discomfort some professionals have with caring for a family experiencing an impending death rather than the typical healthy, live baby.

The same is true for ending a pregnancy. If professionals are not aware of the support that exists and the life consequences that follow, it might show in their body language or the words used. Both paths are painful and extremely hard to traverse, especially when the bomb being dropped is unexpected. It is our wish that while reading this book you will have more insight and stories to share with families early in their journeys. And we hope that you will see and become familiar with the wealth of resources for parents and their families.

IF YOU ARE A PARENT

This is a book written primarily for parents and their families. Most of the time births go well and babies are born healthy. Many women are able to carry their healthy babies to term, take them home from the hospital, love them, care for them, and raise them for a lifetime. This is the norm—every parent's expectation.

However, that childbirth narrative is not what every family experiences, as some parents know all too well. There are far too many parents in this world who have serious and sometimes fatal outcomes, significantly changing their stories and their futures.

Each time a healthy child is born, it is an amazing miracle. Surely, this was also your dream.

However, when things go awry and serious, catastrophic problems are discovered partway through a pregnancy, it is a tragedy of unimaginable proportion. Many parents-to-be are shocked to hear the news that their baby may have a life-threatening disorder, a terrible birth defect, or an issue that is "not compatible" with life. At these vulnerable moments, when hopes and dreams are dashed, parents are overcome with shock and disbelief that they are one of the unlucky ones.

Sadly, you were given such devastating news about your baby or about mom's health that may have even threatened her life. No one can prepare you for such news. Perhaps the baby can survive with disabilities; perhaps the baby will die because of prematurity or due to the problems discovered. In any case, you were probably given little time to make a decision. Either you could continue the pregnancy, waiting for the baby to die on his own, or you could wait to see how severe the problems will be when he finally is born. Or you were asked to agree to terminate the pregnancy, ending the baby's life. In either situation, it was a diagnosis no parent ever wants to hear, and a decision no parent ever wants to make.

> "Your child will not survive. She is not compatible with life. These are your options: you need to think about palliative care or terminate the pregnancy of one of your twins now." I was twenty-six weeks pregnant with my girls. They were both still very much alive inside of me. I was in shock, staring into space, and unable to hold a conversation. Our lives were turned upside down. —Nathalie Himmelrich, mother of twins Ananda Mae and Amya, who died, and author of *Grieving Parents—Surviving Loss As a Couple*

You may have learned the news during routine testing or even at an ultrasound. Your care provider may have had some concerns about you or the baby, which ended with those devastating words. "Your child is not likely to survive or will have life-threatening problems." For some parents, learning that mom has a serious, life-threatening situation such as a placental abruption, organ failure, or other issue that means either both mom and baby will die or baby will die so mom can live feels like a bombshell. The choice is never, ever easy, especially because the life of your baby means everything to you.

If you find this book prior to making such a heartbreaking decision, we want you to know that there are some resources available to help you through that decision: books, experts, doctors, family members, and others who have lived through it. Sherokee has written *Precious Lives, Painful Choices: A Prenatal Decision-making Guide*, which offers immediate, practical help in decision making, along with information about the pros and cons of the two choices. In case you are in immediate need of such resources, this book is also available for download at www.MemoreMedia.com or on Amazon.com. And in case you have not yet terminated your pregnancy, we encourage you to at least read chapter 6, "Birth Plans and Preparation," so that you can utilize some of those ideas for helping you to plan how to meet and be with your baby. Most health care providers do not think to offer such specific planning, which can help you gain control, better prepare, and teach you the importance of making memories and gathering mementos for comfort in the days ahead.

As you read further in this book, we assume you have either ended your wanted pregnancy or are committed to continuing it. By now you have made the decision, even taken the steps and can't or won't go back. We will take you from that point forward. The messages of understanding and hope, along with the quotes and stories included are meant to offer assistance with the realities you may face, the struggles ahead, and the hope that can come when you realize that you are not alone, that others have lived and even thrived—though it may be hard to believe—after such a crisis.

Suddenly being dropped into this position, you know how important it is to find good resources, get connected to helpful people, and know for sure that you are not the only one who has been on this path.

This book includes a wealth of resources that can help you to plan a memorial service, help with other children, find memory items, locate social media support, and more. Within the various chapters of this book, we have purposely included helpful resources to make your journey easier. You will also find a list of resources at the end of the book.

We found that there are precious few resources to help parents *after* such a decision is made—and this book was written to do just that. You will want to know how to live with the aftermath of the tough choice you made (or the decision that was made for you)—to end the pregnancy or to live through a fragile pregnancy. You deserve wise counsel and support as you recover and struggle to live through this bombshell and its aftermath. We know it has radically changed your pregnancy and your life forever.

We each have had babies die, so we intimately know such heartache. We have lived and learned about how to cope over the years since our losses. After meeting, counseling, supporting, and interviewing others who have been in your position, this book is our gift to help you to deal with your present situation and to go forward as positively and as well-informed as possible.

Our hearts go out to you at this time and in the days ahead. We hope you find insight, comfort, support, and hope within these pages.

HOW TO USE THIS BOOK

In this book, we offer you a compelling and practical look at what to consider as you walk your path. You will see that you are not alone. You will see that you share similarities with others who made similar or different decisions—feelings of guilt, questions of faith, concerns about how to talk with others, intense grief responses, the need for support, and so on. However, there are some distinct issues that might be more relevant to you depending upon your path. Therefore, we split the book into three parts. This introduction is meant for all readers. Part I is focused on those who continue their pregnancies, Part II is for those who ended their pregnancies, and Part III is once again intended for all readers. There is no need to read it from beginning to end. Pick the chapters and parts that speak to you. You may read something that might not be helpful to you. Use what you can, dismiss what you wish, then move on. You will notice that we chose to use "he" at times and "she" in other places when referring to your baby rather than "he or she." Take note of the Resources at the end of the book. Though it could never be comprehensive, it is replete with resources to get you started.

Part I focuses on the journey of continuing the pregnancy. In it we walk you through common issues faced by parents who continued their pregnancies. Some of the chapters in this section can also be useful for those who ended a pregnancy but have not yet met their child, such as chapter 6, "Birth Plans and Preparation." We share stories of other parents, tips and advice, and information about the challenges, including how to embrace the pregnancy and even to find joy while carrying your baby. We also hope to help you feel more comfortable as you meet your child and make the most of the time you have. Some topics include how to find specific ideas about being present with your baby during the short time you have her in your life; how to communicate as a couple and interact with others; and how to continue being the parent of your child who has died. We hope you are inspired to create and boldly tell your own child's story.

Part II focuses on the journey after ending the pregnancy. Here you will find information about how to live after such a devastating loss. We offer you help with how to talk with your partner, how to interact with your community, how to cherish your memories, as well as how to move ahead in your healing journey. You will read quotes from and stories about other parents; you will find tips, advice, and lots of resources. How you tell your story to others matters, and how you view it yourself will frame your baby's story and short life. Suggestions are offered for coping with the normal feelings of guilt and blame, along with ways to heal.

Part III is meant to help you continue your healing journey in the weeks, months, and years ahead. It includes common themes of helping your other children, postpartum issues, returning to work, understanding grief and loss, more about men and women, issues for singles, finding support, subsequent pregnancy issues, the possibility of no more babies, and much more.

Both decisions are devastating. There are many similarities but also some very different challenges. No matter which way you go, you have a process ahead that can be lightened with more understanding and compassion. Your extended community will likely question your decision, whatever the decision, and offer you advice. It may feel, or actually be, judgmental, which can add to the pain and feelings of isolation.

We have tried not to inject any personal philosophies or beliefs. Rather, we offer our love and hope to instill the belief that you can make it. You can put your world back together, despite the devastation that this bombshell suddenly dropped on your happy, hopeful life.

DECISIONS MADE AFTER RECEIVING THE NEWS

Having a baby is one of the world's most amazing things. And when all goes well, it is a miracle. Yet for many that miracle is expected, and other outcomes (such as problems with the baby or your health) are not discussed or heard. Pregnancies result in babies, healthy babies, around whom you plan a future full of beautiful dreams. Of course it makes sense. You were expecting good news, not bad. Most babies are born without problems, and that joy is what every mother and father should have. Sadly, the unexpected does happen.

Your world was shattered after this bombshell dropped. An eerie, trancelike shock, followed by a fog of thick debris and dust made it difficult to breathe, to think, or to find clarity about this heartbreaking decision. You were asked to move quickly through the rubble, making a rational, life-altering decision that no parent can ever be prepared to make. You did not choose this. The shock, distress, and confusion hit, and you may still be there, thinking "these things don't happen to babies anymore and they sure couldn't be happening to me." Disbelief is a common reaction; it takes time for the words and meaning to sink in. This is a sign of shock, and a coping mechanism that keeps you from keeling over.

> I remember laughing with my mother, knowing that the doctors had made a mistake. They were looking at me, expecting an answer, and I had none. How could I make a decision about something that I thought would never happen? —Stephanie

Once you came to believe that the diagnosis was possible, or even real, you may find yourself asking the question other parents frequently ask: "What kind of mother (or father) am I?" No parent should have to be in that situation, yet you are. With little time to dwell on this, you probably moved into the information-gathering mode. You may have spent hours on the Internet researching the condition, resources, and organizations. Or maybe someone did that for you. You might have had conversations with your family, faith community, specialists, or others. You might have stayed to yourself, keeping others out of the process, in order to make this intimate decision by yourselves. Or you may have even fallen into a black hole with no way to get out, no words to contribute, no ability to think, let alone to make such a critical decision. This is raw vulnerability. Your protective bubble has burst. Horrible things can happen to good people like you, and now you may even ask, "When will the next shoe drop?" You probably feel weak, defenseless, helpless, and exposed—and in shock.

This may not be your only loss. Maybe you had previous miscarriages or a later loss. You might have even had a previous unexpected prenatal outcome and can't believe it has happened to you again. Expect to feel those other losses resurface. This is unfair and emotionally challenging as other wounds also open up.

> So we interrupted another much-wanted pregnancy at fifteen weeks. The flood of emotions that has occurred has been indescribable, and that neatly tucked away "black box" from two years again resurfaced with a vengeance. I am currently grieving the loss of my second son, but because I never dealt with the emotions from the first, I'm grieving the first loss as well. —B. T.

As you look back on the last few hours or days, maybe you had a foreboding (some mothers do), or maybe not. There are thousands of parents who face this dilemma. They have traveled this heartbreaking road, and they have survived, despite fears they would not. Sharing their hard-earned wisdom is a goal for many, a way for their experience to have meaning and for their child to have a legacy. And that is a goal of this book.

Whether your decision was based on religious or spiritual grounds, moral or ethical considerations, family pressure, mom's health, personal needs and fears, or financial or health reasons, you are not alone.

In *Precious Lives, Painful Choices: A Prenatal Decision-making Guide*, Ilse asks, "which decision will be the one that you can live with the best? The one that will haunt you the least. The one that seems less hard (but, of course, is never easy)." As you faced this overwhelming dilemma, you made the best choice for you and your beloved child, given the little you know right now. Hopefully, you can now work on moving ahead.

> None of the choices offered were my choices. I hated that word. It's like asking someone to willingly choose which prison they'd like to go to for the next thirty years. There is no joy, not a good choice at all. I would never choose either of them. —Vicki Culling, *Holding On & Letting Go*

Maybe you are in the early days after the decision to continue your pregnancy or maybe you are further along. If you ended your pregnancy, we assume you have already delivered your baby and have said good-bye. In any case, now there is more for you to do and consider. How you move forward matters. There is a community of caring people who want to help you to do this with the fewest regrets and the most support.

There are so many uncertainties you probably will consider:

- What if we made the wrong choice?
- How do we talk about it to our family and community?
- What if we made a choice that goes against our own beliefs or our faith community's beliefs?
- Will our baby experience any pain?
- Will our baby feel and know our love?
- Will our baby die in peace?
- Will others question our decision and judge us?
- What will they say to us and what do we say to them?
- Where do we go next? We feel stuck and unable to move; how do we go forward?
- Are we the only ones? Have others survived?
- If our baby survives what will be her quality of life?
- When our baby dies after the procedure, what are our rights to meet him and claim his body for our final good-byes?

You deserve some help with these questions in the days ahead. You'll find discussions about many of these points in the following chapters. They are also good questions to ask your medical caregiver.

With all of this uncertainty, confusion, and heartache, many parents feel it is not survivable—not just for your baby, but for both parents. You ache deep within your heart and soul. You probably want to turn back the clock and have your innocence back. Most parents feel this. You are not alone.

FINDING LIGHT AFTER THE DARKNESS

You may wonder if you will ever smile again, laugh out loud, and be positive and hopeful. It is common to have concerns that you will live a life of fear, regret, and sadness. Healing from such an event takes much work and lots of mourning over time, which can feel like forever. But it is evident from stories and studies that virtually all parents in your situation come out the other end—never to forget, of course. Hopefully you find solace and comfort from others who care and understand. And if you do your personal grief work, you can—and we believe you will—survive and hopefully thrive in the future. However, a piece of your heart will be missing as you remember your child who is no longer physically present. You will need no reminders from others that you forever will be the parent of this baby.

You will be challenged to find ways to incorporate your child into your life as you go forward. Parents are always parents, even if their child died before them. Parenting a child who becomes only a memory—although a very important person nonetheless—takes creativity and experimentation. Learn from others about how they keep their children alive in their hearts. Each child holds a place in the family and cannot, nor should not, be forgotten.

In *Holding On & Letting Go* (2013), Vicki Culling credits the "power of parents' stories to help in feeling less alone and in healing. Stories of continuing and stories of letting go shed light on the many questions and concerns that parents naturally have. They also can offer assurance of finding hope and help." *A Gift of Time: Continuing Your Pregnancy When Your Baby's Life Is Expected to Be Brief* (2011) is another book full of such stories and advice from parents who continued their pregnancies. *Our Heartbreaking Choices: Forty-six Women Share Their Stories of Interrupting a Much-Wanted Pregnancy* (2008) by Christie Brooks offers stories for those who ended their pregnancies.

What story do you tell to those close to you and to new people you meet? How have you changed and what matters to you now? There can be many special moments and shared experiences with others during this journey as you retell your child's story over the years. It need not be only hardship and pain. Your baby brought you joy, hope, and mostly love. Remember that. Be open to feeling that love and the specialness of your baby, no matter the problems and the struggles. Parents repeatedly tell us that they changed in profound and beautiful ways as a result of the time they spent with their babies. Seek that light, which may not come right away and may not stay very long in the early days. With an open attitude and heart, you can feel it and find it when ready. Embrace those gifts and recognize the light that shines even in the darkness.

QUESTIONING ONE'S FAITH

It is easy to feel overwhelmed and in deep shock and anguish. This news cuts you off at the knees. How will you make it through? Are you one who believes in God, or do you believe that you can handle this yourself? Do you have a community who gives you the strength you need to go forward during tough times? Or do you feel small, helpless, and alone? What role does faith and belief in a greater being play in your life? At times like these, people often feel either drawn to God and faith or pushed away.

As an imperfect human being, you may wonder how you will make it through the pregnancy or, alternatively, how you will make it through the aftermath of the termination. Where will you find your strength and courage? Asking for help and desperately needing strong support can make you feel vulnerable and lonely.

How does a loving God allow this to happen to good people? Many parents share how much they prayed for the health of their babies only to find their prayers did not keep their babies safe and healthy. Anger at God or the universe is a natural outcry from pain and fear, as are feelings of abandonment. On the other hand, some people live with the belief that they are not in control and that when things happen—bad or good—it will work out in the end. And still others do not believe in a God, yet may still have a similar outcry.

When bad things happen, many look to their faith, to their God. You may ask for a miracle through prayer. You may ask others to pray for you and that miracle. You may feel that you have been deeply let down. Why didn't you get good news instead of bad? You may wonder what you did wrong to cause this. Looking for a cause and feeling out of control are normal reactions to such horrific news and the path that you now find yourself on. After all, you may have a strong faith or belief that you are a good person and that such things should not be happening to you and your family.

If you have questions, if you feel your faith is challenged, or if you are seeking a closer relationship with God in order to live through this, go to your faith advisers, to prayer, to the Bible, Torah, or whatever fits your religious beliefs, and to the people who surround you. Find those who can listen while you talk through your questions, confusion, pain, and hope.

> As I traveled down the dark highway in an ambulance to the hospital, He held me under His wings ever so tightly and whispered, "Be not afraid." I knew the Lord held both my baby and I that night. But I was afraid after that this was the end for my nineteen-week son. Now was the time to cling to the substance of things hoped for, Father, that beautiful and gentle word. —Jennifer Ross, *Isaiah's Story*

Explaining why this has happened and why prayers for miracles may seem fruitless is not something we can answer. What we want to do is to affirm that you have the right to these feelings, that it is hard to go through this alone. Many of us have found love and understanding that has given us guidance and strength to endure, no matter the choice, no matter the path.

Maybe you do not have a strong faith in God or other spiritual being. Your strengths and sources of support come from other places. Maybe you find calm in meditation or nature. Or maybe you have counselors and friends who guide you and help hold you up. Whatever has worked in the past may also work now, or you may wish to explore other avenues. Even if you feel incredibly lonely and fall into the depths of despair (common responses), remember there is help out there and you are not the only one.

There are many Christian parents who find comfort knowing that God allowed his only son, Jesus, to die for the sins of others. What pain that must have been for God! Many do come to believe that He knows the pain of having a child die and is there to offer comfort and understanding. This message may come straight to you from reading His word, or from others who are there to care for you.

> I was so angry with God when we were told our son could die and we were asked to choose a time for his death or carry him for months before he would die. How could a loving God do this to us? Why were we not spared from this disaster? Then someone very dear told me that God knows the pain of having a child suffer and die; He would never purposely put that upon anyone. Rather, He is there to hold us up and offer understanding and grace throughout our time of loss and grief. Most days that is enough to help me get through the day. There are still times I wonder, but thankfully, I do believe this and it rights my path and touches my heart. —A mom

Some parents don't ask "Why me?"; they ask "Why *not* me?" In the randomness of life, what makes someone so special that bad things don't happen to him or her? You may be one who thinks like this. Maybe other terrible things have happened to you, and you aren't surprised when lightning strikes again. Whether you understand that suffering comes to everyone or you feel the victim of too many painful challenges, your attitude makes a difference in how you cope. If you look for the positives in life, keep doing that now. There are many who get through tragedies like this with a better attitude than others.

> After we learned our daughter had Potter's Syndrome, we did not ask "Why us?" but "Why not us?" Are we exempt from suffering while there are so many who suffer significant hardships themselves? We found things to be thankful for—the kind caregivers, the fact that we both had jobs and health insurance, and that we had some family members who were present for us. We chose to turn to God in our darkest moments. And we realized that our situation could be much worse. —A mom

If you are angry at God or the universe, let it out. Express it and share it, which can help you better understand your feelings. Others who may have also had such struggles can also be of help. Trust that in time you will regain your balance and find your source of strength. Blessings and grace may very well come upon you in most unusual and interesting ways. Open your heart to consider if faith can help you endure and eventually thrive as you find your new normal and keep your baby alive in your heart and within your family.

However, if turning to God for support is not something you can do now, even if you have been a faith-filled person, give it time. Pray for guidance and seek spiritual support from clergy and others who have these beliefs and share their wisdom well.

GUILT, BLAME, AND SHAME

Guilt and Regret

There are many reasons why people have feelings of guilt about the various choices they made when faced with a poor fetal diagnosis. Many feel they did something wrong to deserve such bad news. Others feel guilt about terminating a wanted pregnancy. Still others may feel guilt about carrying an unhealthy baby to term, only to die very shortly thereafter or to live a longer but physically limited life. And many parents through the years have shared that they felt guilt about the decision they made.

Guilt is one of the most common and universal feelings, which can be caused by an action or event or by nothing at all. Each day we all find things that we wish we had done differently or that we feel guilty about. It is a human condition. Most people seek to do the right thing. Although we are not perfect, we wish that we could live without mistakes and regrets, that we could make the right decisions in every situation.

If something bad happens, most of us want to understand what went wrong and what could be changed in the future. We replay it in our minds, trying to imagine what would have happened if we had done things differently. Most people with children who have serious problems or with pregnancy complications have deep feelings of guilt. This seems especially true for moms who feel that they may have caused the problem. Fathers can also have feelings of guilt. What part might they have played? These are natural, human reactions to disappointment and tragedy. All moms and dads want and plan for healthy newborns. Although you might have had concerns or fears that something could go wrong, it was not the dream you held.

After all, as mothers, we are told to take care of ourselves and our babies—drink lots of water, take folic acid and vitamins, exercise, pay attention to the baby's movements, obtain prenatal care, and avoid alcohol and too much coffee, and more. If we are the protectors of our babies, how do we feel when they are not healthy or might die? Like most mothers in this situation, you will look back on what you did, what you ate, how you cared for yourself, and even your emotions and thoughts. In virtually all situations, there is nothing that you could have done differently. On one level, you can make sense of that. But on another level, as the mother-protector, it doesn't seem quite right. Surely something could have been done differently. And if you discover something that you think could be a possible cause, you may keep it secreted inside or share it with a few people. Again, this is very normal; many mothers admit to having such feelings. Rarely is there proof that something you did caused the baby's problems or impending death. But that doesn't mean those feelings will go away easily, despite their irrationality. Don't let it eat away at you. Do your research, be open to the idea that things can happen despite your best efforts, and if you still can't let those feelings go, try to give yourself grace and forgiveness.

You may fear that your partner blames you or even feel you have reasons why he could blame you. Again, though these are probably irrational thoughts and unlikely causes, they still may be inside eating away at you. Feeling guilty that things went wrong in the pregnancy or with mom's body makes sense; it just doesn't help much. Feeling guilty that you couldn't do anything about it also makes sense, but it does not change anything. Looking for someone to blame is also another natural response.

Since you are likely reading this book after making your decision, it is appropriate to also talk about the guilt that can arise as a result of the decision you made. Or the decision was made for you, for reasons such as serious health concerns for mom, or even because you learned of your baby's problems late in the pregnancy and are on a path for delivery with no real options. Second-guessing is natural. When the bombshell was dropped and your world was shattered, you were given little time and perhaps few resources to make a good decision. And even if you made the best decision you could given the circumstances, you may still feel guilt and regret because it was a decision you never would have made if not put in that position, through no fault of your own. You are not the only one feeling this kind of doubt, guilt, and regret. If you visit some of the social media sites or sit in a room with others who are where you are, this would be the primary point of conversation. We have heard it often. Indeed, you are not alone. And no one can take those feelings away. You must find a way to deal with them by doing such things as sharing, writing, seeking counseling, praying, forgiving, and healing.

> I know this is the decision we had to make at the time. But now that we have had more time to do research and really think about it, I regret the decision. And I feel so guilty. My husband is not quite there, but I can tell he has second thoughts. Why did we have to decide so quickly? Why didn't we do more research and talk with others who had been there, too? We can't go back, but I wish we could. I feel so guilty and cry all the time. —A mom, shared in a support group

We made it. We own it. We will live with it. Period. —A father, shared in a support group

Shame and Self-blame

Shame and self-blame are also common feelings held by parents who feel that they created a less-than-perfect child. Other people have healthy babies, you may think, "What did we do that caused our baby to be unhealthy?" Many expectant mothers describe themselves as failures. Even if you have other living children, you can still feel like you failed with this child. Shame is a common childhood feeling that often carries into adulthood. Just because you grew up and matured does not mean shameful feelings disappear. They may resurface at times like this. Of course, this is understandable. The baby was growing inside mom and something went wrong. Where does the blame go? For many, it goes inside and hurts deeply. Shame disables many people from sharing their experiences with others. It may keep you from reaching out to others who might be helpful or who just want to be there for you. If you are ashamed about how things turned out, others might sense that and think you don't want or need their help. Yet most people are very sympathetic to the loss of an unborn child or to the birth of a disabled or unhealthy child.

There is no shame in the outcome of your pregnancy. Most birth defects or problems are no one's fault. However, dealing with those feelings is important, and talking to a professional, whether your ob-gyn, a trained and licensed counselor, or a member of the clergy, may help you to handle these emotions. Discussing your feelings with your partner or others may help you. Old stigmas have been replaced by new information about prenatal health, and talking about losses and poor diagnoses is more often met nowadays with compassion, understanding, and friendship.

A mom we spoke with relayed her story to us about how she came to help a friend with a poor prenatal diagnosis:

> Our first child had trisomy 18 thirteen years ago. We opted to induce labor at about twenty-three weeks and our son was stillborn. I didn't discuss it widely, not for any particular reason. No one I knew had gone through it, and while many were sympathetic about our loss, no one really understood the choice we made. Years later, in another

town where we moved, a neighbor—just an acquaintance at the time—reported being pregnant with twins. I had just had twins of my own, my third and fourth children, and we became a little closer discussing what raising twins was like—these would be her fourth and fifth children. A few weeks later, she e-mailed the entire neighborhood to report she'd lost one of the twins, but that she was fine, the other baby was fine, and she didn't feel the need to dwell on it. I took a breath and wrote her back, detailing how our first had died. I explained most of the details and how difficult it had been for us at the time to have had a child die so far along. She was about sixteen weeks when this happened to her, and she wrote back to me that, in fact, the one twin also had trisomy 18, and her growth would have endangered the other healthier twin. They chose to terminate, but she was devastated, despite her earlier insistence that she was fine. By reaching out to her, I was able to talk further with her about her feelings—and mine!—and we became fast and close friends. She felt so ashamed of her decision, so worried it was the wrong one, but together we could talk about those feelings and work through them. It's years later now, and her son is healthy and thriving. She and I are both done having children, but we never forget the ones who died.
—Anonymous

Blaming Others

If you don't blame your body and wonder what you did that might have caused this, then you may ask, "Well, who is to blame?" If it turns out to be a genetic problem that's inherited, another round of doubt and self-blame can occur, and you may blame your partner or your ancestors. There is plenty of blame to go around when something so heartbreaking happens. It's important to remember in these moments that our biology is not our fault. We are born with certain traits and genes that give us our hair color, our skin tone, and our height, but some babies inherit other genes that may take a wrong turn for them. We don't choose our genes. We don't choose our ancestors. It may help in these cases to discuss your worries further with a genetic counselor, who can reassure you and explain what factors go into these outcomes for unborn children.

You may feel betrayed by your medical caregiver or find the way they gave you the news to be upsetting (this is a very common complaint that compounds the tough pain you are in). You may blame them for putting you on a testing roller coaster without adequately explaining that once the information is known, it can't be unknown. Most parents-to-be do not realize that once they learn the results, they may be put in a position where a decision must be made about going forward with the pregnancy or not.

"Why did I ever take the tests?" you may wonder. Maybe you agreed without fully understanding the serious consequences of hearing anything less than good news. Maybe you gladly took the test feeling invincible, hoping that all would be just fine. Or maybe you had some doubts and sought reassurance, hoping the tests would provide the security you needed.

As a result, you went through extra testing, heard devastating news, and then had to actually make a life-altering, unimaginable decision. If you had known all this, maybe you wouldn't have taken the tests in the first place. Maybe you would rather have had a blissful, enjoyable pregnancy and would have dealt with whatever happened at the end. In any case, this type of blame is quite normal. You may wish you could rewind the tape and go back. Sadly, you cannot. It's okay to have feelings of blame and even anger as long as they don't hurt you (or others) more. Own them and realize that you have the choice to let them harm you and others or not. There are many choices you will need to make on this journey. Your attitude and behaviors are something you can work on. Write them down, share them with others, see a counselor, or find a support person or group online. Just don't let your feelings overtake you.

Regrets about Your Decision

At times you may question the choice you made. This is another common theme shared by parents in your situation. Although you may regret the path you took—something many parents say—it is behind you. You did the best you could at the time with what you knew. Now you need to find ways to go forward positively as you deal with the new circumstances.

Just know that these feelings are normal and not surprising. Many question their choices and regret their decisions. It could be a trip that is planned when something horrible happens, a doctor who is selected to care for your child who causes your child unnecessary suffering, a job change that turns out to be worse than the previous job, a move to another home or community that turns into a disaster. Regrets occur in life.

The question to ask is, Will these regrets define you and control you? Or will you work to keep them in check and understand that you did not choose this. You wanted this baby and you would never have imagined such an outcome. You do not have to become the person who is buried in these feelings. You can work to free yourself so that you can go forward using healthy grieving strategies.

> It took me years to get beyond daily guilt. There was a lot of repeating to myself, "there was nothing that I could do." —Jennifer

While it is normal and acceptable to have these feelings, you may wish you had ideas for things to do to deal with and counter such intense emotions. There are many things you can do to take the focus from them and to find or make some positives in your life.

One mother shared the following, "After our first son died, I spent a lot of time doing creative things—making little bits of 'art' that I still keep around my house. They aren't very good (I'm no artist), but they remind me of that time and how I passed it. Also, I sought counseling at one point, though it wasn't a good fit. I spent time with good friends and treated myself often (to new clothes and ice cream, etc.). I bought my husband a small $4 ivy plant; we've grown it for thirteen years and still tend it! It helps me feel like we're still taking care of our child in some small way."

TIPS AND ADVICE

- Repeat to yourself, "I did the best I could at the time with what I knew." Now find ways to go forward positively as you deal with the new circumstances.
- Bring your inner feelings and worries to the outside, literally. Write down what you feel guilty about and why (if you know). Write down who you blame and why. Then think about the word shame to see if it is something you are carrying in your heart. Write this word down or simply say it out loud and any reasons why you feel shame. Now

you can share them with someone (a dear friend or a counselor) or tuck them away in your private journal. You could also tear them up or burn them while asking your baby, your God, or yourself for forgiveness and love.

- Talk with your partner about feelings you each may have. Although you can't take them away from each other, you can show your love and support. Help one another think about how painful and harsh these feelings are. Ask yourselves if they are helping you or hurting you more.

- Imagine that you are releasing balloons with a note attached. What words do you need to rid from your mind, body, and soul? If you were to write them and release them into the clouds, how might you feel? One mother shared that the words she kept repeating to herself were destructive (bad mother, angry at doctor, angry at self, failure, unlovable, frustration). After releasing them, she felt her self-inflicted load on her heart had been relieved. Then write the words that feel good and give you power and positive feelings, words such as lovable, good mother, did my best, grateful, and hopeful. Tuck them into your mind and your pocket.

- Tell yourself that feelings of guilt, shame, self-blame, and blaming others are real, understandable, and what makes you human. Then ask yourself if you think these feelings are getting in the way of what you need to do right now. Are they feelings you want to keep? Or can you let them lighten up or go away? They are yours and only you can decide whether they will build nests in your hair or will fly away (an old Chinese proverb).

- Make time for lighthearted activities, if you can. Create things (woodworking, home projects, needlepoint, knitting, beading, sewing, ceramics, etc.). You can find a sense of rebirth and satisfaction after a small or large project is complete.

- Help others, even in small ways. Make a meal for a sick friend, donate funds to a favorite charity in your child's name, or participate in a run, walk, or other fundraiser for a good cause.

HOW TO TELL OTHERS

Although you may wish that you could hibernate in the early days and weeks after your loss, you may realize that you can't. You live in a community of family, work colleagues, a neighborhood, and perhaps a faith community. It is inevitable that you will be around people far sooner than you may wish. Interacting with others in the early days following your decision can be stressful. Soon after learning the news of your baby's diagnosis, you may have to let some of your close family and friends know what is going on, but most probably do not know. Some might have helped guide you during that difficult decision-making time. Others might have offered to support you through the pregnancy. And if you ended the pregnancy, others may have been there to support you during the procedure or birth. There may be some who stepped away, afraid and unaware of how to help you. They are uncomfortable or confused about how to respond.

Whether you are scared and worried about the decision or feel that it was a clear and necessary choice, you may wonder how others will respond. One of the hardest things may be to tell others. Most people will ask questions because they are naturally curious and because they want to help you. However, given the circumstances, the pressures of society, and the reality that there are people who question why you would continue an abnormal pregnancy or who do not support ending a pregnancy for any reason, you may be concerned about how the news will be received. That is reality. There will also be some who respond positively. They may be able to get beyond their own concerns and beliefs because they know you are hurting and need love and care. Friends and family will be in shock and will feel some of your pain. Unless they have had personal or professional experience with this type of situation, they may not know what to say or do to help. As the news spreads, you will realize that it is a shock for your whole community. The bombshell has hit them, too. They were so happy for you and many had already come to love your baby and to dream of your bright, happy future. Now all will experience loss, something few are comfortable handling.

Consider making sure that your close family and friends are told first. If it is at all possible, share the news in person, which gives them a chance to give you the love and support directly, rather than over the phone. You could ask them to come to your home, rather than meeting in a public place. If not in your home, ask one of your parents or siblings to host a small gathering over tea or dinner. For those who are far away, you could use Skype or FaceTime, so that you can see each other. Or you could make phone calls. To avoid repeating the story, you may want help telling others. Find someone you trust—a parent, a sibling, or a grandparent—whom you can ask to call others, the next "ring" of people. Be careful about doing this; you'll want to make sure that they are relaying the same message to everyone. If you only want to share parts of the story for now, you'll want to cover that in your message.

You may even decide that there are people you won't tell immediately, such as a grandmother who lives far away or work colleagues. It may be that you need to get yourself together and do more research as you figure out what to actually tell them.

Social Media

When it comes to telling people, many naturally turn toward social media. Be very careful about what you write there. You might be surprised both by how much support you receive and by things that some people say, which can cause even more pain. Pause and think it through before you or others post your personal story. There are disadvantages that can cause more drama than you need right now. Although this may be a way to tell many, you might be surprised by some of the responses. Some parents choose to use CaringBridge instead or to tell everyone to go silent on all social media outlets.

If you decide you want to keep the news away from social media, you will want to include this in any messages you or others give out. You can tell your community to keep this news off social media, as it is private and your news to share or not to share. Or you can have a private group where you carefully screen people to minimize the hurtful comments.

We were very open on Facebook, so telling our story of continuing the pregnancy seemed natural. What a mistake. While some friends were truly kind and compassionate, others were not. Two people made rude and upsetting comments. One asked why anyone would go ahead with a pregnancy when the baby would die anyway. She even insinuated that this would harm our other children. The other said that she did not understand why doctors would let a mother continue her pregnancy under these conditions. Both hurt us deeply. We deleted the comments and unfriended them, but the damage had been done. Now we are more careful about what we put on Facebook of a personal and emotional nature. —A mom

There were a few people on Facebook who were rude and hurtful. Even though we didn't put out the whole story, they came to that conclusion. Then they beat us up like crazy. I didn't realize people could be so hurtful. The drama is more than I can take. I highly advise people to be careful, and I wish I had asked everyone to keep things to themselves. *No Facebook!* —A mom

When crafting a message to share—whether via letter, phone call, e-mail, or even social media—consider what you wish others to know and what you wish to keep to yourself. If you don't give out enough information, you can be sure that people will ask questions.

What to Say if You Are Continuing the Pregnancy

If you are continuing the pregnancy, you could say something like, "Our baby is likely to die and we have chosen to let nature take its course. We'll carry the pregnancy until she is born, and we'll take things as they come. At this point, we are busy and overwhelmed; we aren't able to provide more information than that. We'd appreciate your support and prayers."

Here are some other ideas of what you might say as you give the news and ask for support. Be clear so it doesn't leave them guessing. For example, "We are in need of people who trust us right now—friends who do not question our decision and who also love this baby for who he is, no matter what the birth outcome will be." Or you could something in writing such as, "We were shocked to learn that our baby has a serious physical problem that may result in his death or a life of hardship. Our doctor asked us whether we would continue the pregnancy or end the life of our child. We made the difficult but firm decision to be with our baby for the rest of the pregnancy, until his time comes. We still hold out hope that he may yet live and would appreciate your positive thoughts and prayers. There is much we don't yet know, so we will be tied up with medical appointments, research, and preparation. In addition, we want to make the most of our time left with our son. So please understand if we don't keep you fully informed. Rather than having everyone ask questions or be afraid to ask questions, we will use CaringBridge (a free website for such situations) or mass e-mails to communicate when we can. Thank you for your love and understanding."

What to Say if You Have Ended the Pregnancy

One mom wrote, "There are problems with the baby and I prefer not to talk about them right now." You could say, "Our baby died. She had serious problems and was not destined to live." Or "She was born prematurely and did not make it." If you prefer offering more details, you could say, "After testing, we learned early in our pregnancy that our sweet baby might not survive long after birth. He would be in immense pain requiring many surgeries. Therefore, we were asked to do what no parent ever wants to do—save him from that life by ending our pregnancy early. We are in deep pain and hope that you will support us, not judge us."

> I have actually not told many, just those closest to me (four friends and family)—unfortunately in my community it is a very taboo subject, and I am a fairly private person, so I've just left them as miscarriages. I also did not tell very many people we were expecting (both times). My sister told people for me at sixteen weeks with my first son (she was thrilled for me) and only those closest to us knew of my second son. I actually had asked my husband if we could just not tell anyone until we were twenty weeks but he said I would start to show before that. —B.

> I didn't know what to tell people so I avoided the conversation totally. Then I heard from my sister that people were saying all kinds of things, including some crazy things. Clearly, they did not know what happened and what we were going through. I wish I had pushed myself to either write a note to people or tell a dependable relative to spread the word. —A dad

HOW OTHERS RESPOND

How people respond to your news will differ depending on circumstances. After hearing some form of the truth, most people may be uncomfortable and might fumble for words or act as if they didn't hear you. Avoidance and changing the subject are common responses.

Others will approach you and ask awkward questions. For instance, the clerk at the supermarket may inquire about your baby belly, wondering when you are due (even though you may have already had your baby) or about your baby's sex or health. If you share details of your story, she might then focus on your change and bagging the groceries, avoiding eye contact. With no time to prepare how to respond, she likely doesn't know what to do with this surprising and sad news. You may react with intense emotions of pain, loneliness, or even anger for what seems like a lack of care. Or you may take it in stride. After a few such encounters, you may find inner strength to deal with it or you may be hurt each time. Another option is to say nothing in response to the question. You could start digging in your purse or change the subject by asking a question about something unrelated. The more you can go with the flow and lower your stress, the more emotionally and physically healthier you will be.

On the other hand, people may surprise you. Strangers and close friends may be curious, supportive, and affirming after hearing such news. It may be that they have had their own losses or know someone else who has. You won't know how people will respond to your news until you are in that situation. They may show you through their responses and actions that they are on your team. Keep those people close to you.

> We had a lot of support over the following few months but after a while people seemed to move on and not really want to talk about him as it's too painful. But even though there is pain, he is still our son and we never want him forgotten. —Emma

> After too many store clerks and passersby asked me if this was my first, when I was due, and was it a boy or girl, I changed my response from one of being defensive and worried about what to say. Instead, I would say, "Our loved baby is a girl and we cherish every minute with her." That was usually enough, and while not a lie, it offered a

bit of a diversion while I shared my heart without all the details. —A mom

When People Disappear

There will be people who are not able to be there for you and who may "disappear." You may be okay with keeping a distance to minimize the hurt. It is possible that they don't have the courage to face you, they are afraid they will fail or hurt you more, or they have their own hurts and baggage that have now come to the surface. If you need to, let them go. We can also promise you that if you attend support groups or find others like you online or in your community, you will discover good friends who understand you and will stand by you. This is how life goes. We rarely carry our entire community of friends with us throughout our lives. Yes, some may be there always, but the rest come and go. Think about it. This might help you prepare for the new ones and more easily let go of those who need to move on. For more on building community support, read chapter 17, "Building Support from Others."

1

The Journey of Continuing the Pregnancy

You and your partner chose to continue the pregnancy, even though the baby's condition is fatal or life limiting. This takes courage and love, since you know the days and weeks ahead will have many challenges. You may feel relief that at least you won't be the one to choose the day or the time of your baby's death. And now you are expected to go forward in some normal manner, still pregnant, yet no longer innocent.

You are on the path to carry your beloved baby to birth, come what may. Since this is probably new for you, you may wonder where you go next. Concerns and questions may be swirling around your head as you wade through the fog of shock and disbelief that can last a long time. There are so many things to think about: What do you say to others? How do you approach the rest of your pregnancy? Do you have the courage and strength to go forward? Do you even dare go out of the house knowing how complicated it will be when you meet friends and strangers? Are you the only one who has been through such a traumatic pregnancy? How do you find others? What will labor and delivery be like? Might you be at a higher risk for a caesarean? What resources might you need? Consult with your care provider about such lingering concerns.

You and your partner may be on different wavelengths at times and struggle as a couple. On the other hand, you may be in sync and feel you are in agreement as a strong team as you go forward. It is possible that you may be able to experience your child to the fullest, act out your parenting role, and share with others who are supportive. This could be the most powerful experience of your life.

Some parents pray for a miracle and hope that their babies might yet live or might not have severe medical problems after all. While this is not likely to happen often, there are times when it has, and you may hear those stories. Some parents need to hold onto hope; if this is something you need to do, then you will do that. This is your journey and you will follow your own path despite what others say. Other parents might accept what they see as the "inevitable" and once some shock wears off, they begin to seek information and to make plans.

It is natural to have doubts or second thoughts about your decision, along with fears and questions. You cannot see the future and you cannot change the past. There are so many unknowns, and this road is not one you have traveled before. However, as you go forward with your pregnancy and commit your heart to *being* with your baby for as long as you can, you will probably become more secure in this path.

Through it all, remember that your baby is loved by you, your partner, and others. Always rely on and remember this love as you make decisions and memories. Your time together is precious. Be as wise and as open as you can. Focus less on the prognosis and final outcome you fear. Although information seeking and planning must be done, don't let that get in the way of being present. Be your child's parent. Be fully engaged in the time you *do* have together. Making the most of this time is up to you.

> I just want to encourage any women out there to take a palliative care approach to their pregnancy. I did so seven months ago and welcomed my beautiful daughter into the world for one very precious hour. Keep loving your little one and cherishing those little kicks and any other special little interactions between you and your baby. Your time together is now! —Alice

I

EMBRACE YOUR PREGNANCY

LEARNING ABOUT YOUR BABY

How you look at your pregnancy since the diagnosis has likely changed significantly. Chances are that you have or will spend considerable time doing research, going to medical appointments, reading books, blogs, and other Internet sites, and seeking others who have been down this road before. All this, plus working and keeping up your home, job, and family can keep you very busy. At times you may feel like sticking your head under a pillow in hopes that the nightmare will be over. A mom who had a recent loss shares this sentiment with you, "Do not isolate yourself; there are many people in your corner—those who have 'been there, done that' and also those who have not had a loss and want to support you."

Feeling overwhelmed and stuck is common in the early hours. You may feel alone and may not have anyone to turn to who can offer guidance, but when you find that person, so much can change. You will have help breaking things down into small steps and decisions, one at a time.

Despite it all, you may recognize immediately that you want to embrace the time you have with your baby since you no longer have a lifetime to embrace one another. Mom, you are the nurturer (unless you break stereotype and dad is), so give in to your nurturing self as you go through this pregnancy one day at a time.

One of the more important things parents consistently say is that they slowly came to understand that they needed to make the most of the precious time they had with their baby. You may also realize that this is the only time you'll be all together. Even if it is weeks or months, it will be too short, yet it can be made special and memorable. Experience your child to the fullest, making precious memories that will give you comfort over time. However, you may be full of fear about living through the pregnancy and seeing your child. What will he look like? Will the deformities be more than you can bear to see? The anxiety and list of fears may be piling up, which is quite understandable.

My baby was diagnosed with multiple fetal anomalies, and I don't think they are related. I think each one is its own rare disease, which adds more confusion to my pain as to why this could be happening. My eyes are so swollen from crying and I am so tired. I want to sleep, but when I do, it's just nightmares. I wake up with night tremors and have panic attacks. This is killing me, yet it's my baby who is dying.
—Anonymous

The ultrasound report at fourteen weeks listed the following terms: Encephalocele; Skeletal Dysplasia; Fetal Hydrops; Thanatophoric Dwarfism. I would appreciate your comments and advice, because you can trigger me to think about things I need to think about and not push off or ignore. For example, how do I handle my other children about this (ages five, three, and one)? The problem I am thinking about now is I can barely deal with the pregnancy, how am I going to look at this baby? The way the doctors explained, he is so deformed and I just picture a monster in my dreams. I don't know. It's all really just overwhelming —Toni-Marie in an e-mail to Sherokee

One dad spoke this profound and honest thought, "It didn't take us long to make our decision. We knew he deserved to live the rest of his life, no matter how long or short that was. But then we had to live through many months of hell. What a feeling of powerlessness as a father who can't do anything." It was a period of intense grief as they awaited the birth of their son and they couldn't fix his problems.

Yes, this is overwhelming and surely not the way you dreamed about it. But does it need to be that bad every week and every day? Do you think you can seek some joy and share your love as you take your baby with you shopping, to weddings, to church, to synagogue, to work, on a date with your partner, and to family events? Your attitude can make all the difference (even if you choose to fake it sometimes). This is the time you get together.

FRUSTRATION WITH MEDICAL CARE PROVIDERS

You may carry pain and upset feelings due to words medical professionals or others used when talking with you, words such as "incompatible with life," "termination," "interruption," "fetus," "abortion," "late-term abortion," "medical abortion," and "products of conception." These words were not used to intentionally hurt you. Despite protests of many parents, medical jargon is not easy to change. Although words and conversations may haunt you at times, make some choices. You can choose to disavow or ignore those words and to use your own words. This is your son or daughter. If you have a name for your baby, say it. Decide not to dwell on those negative feelings if possible. Instead, give your attention to one another, your baby, and any other children you might already have. When and if you feel up to it, let your caregivers know what their medical terms mean to you. Perhaps at an appointment or some other point down the road, you could tell them your concerns. If you have ideas for how they could have done it better, tell them or try writing it down in a diary or journal and moving on.

MAKE THE MOST OF YOUR TIME TOGETHER

As you move ahead, you will have good days. Embrace and appreciate them. And you will have bad and hard days. Understand and accept them. Focus for a moment on the fact that you are still pregnant and your baby is still alive. Take it one step at a time. Don't allow all of your worries to overwhelm you. Instead, consider one or two concerns at a time.

You may wonder how you actually make the most of it. Love your baby, as you would any child. Start there. Your situation and the path you have chosen now offers you the chance to continue to get to know your child and to embrace each moment you have together. Your child knows your voice, your love, and probably your dreams. Do what you can to put your fears and worries aside, even if for a few hours each day in the beginning. Your baby is still safe and warm inside you, mom. You'll have years to grieve and miss your child; that is inevitable. It is important to do your best to make the remaining time with your baby to be treasured and filled with love. This is how you experience and share, in a positive way, the next weeks and months as a family.

In *Waiting with Gabriel*, mother Amy Kuebelbeck set a high bar for the time she had left with her son after receiving a fatal diagnosis at five and a half months of pregnancy. She, her husband, and their two children did everything they could with Gabriel. While still pregnant, they took him to the zoo, on picnics, on family trips, and so much more as a means of showing love and experiencing the special time they had left with him. She also cowrote another book, *A Gift of Time*, with Deborah L. Davis. This book shares stories and specific advice about how parents made the most of the time with their babies, what they regretted, and why they were grateful. The depth of stories can certainly provide guidance and help you feel less alone. Amy has joined others to advocate for a supportive system of palliative care also called perinatal hospice programs that help families live through their pregnancies, make plans, and be supported at the time of birth, death, or during the life of special needs babies, and beyond. She also has a powerful, resource-rich website, www.perinatalhospice.org, as well as her website, www.waitingwithgabriel.com.

Sophia's parents decided to do everything they could to celebrate her life while pregnant with her, knowing that it was likely she would die before birth. They wanted a baby shower and asked everyone to give their favorite book. Over the course of many months, they read each book to Sophia. They also read her stories of miracles from the Bible every night. Sophia's mom Stephanie would tell Andy, Sophia's father, every time Sophia kicked so that he could revel in it. Clearly, they made the most of a terrible situation by being present and celebratory as often as possible. Prior to birth they had her baptized, knowing that at that moment she was still alive. They are grateful they could carry this attitude into the birth and beyond. They created a twelve-minute YouTube video to share with others living through such a pregnancy.

"We had a lot of laughs with her," Stephanie said about talking to her baby Sophia in pregnancy. "She was a little prankster. And sometimes I'd ask, 'Sophia, are you still here?' She always gave me the answer with a kick."

Include Family

It is easy to get caught up in your needs as a couple and to focus on how to include your other children. However, it is appropriate and wise to invite your extended family, especially grandparents, to join you in making the most of this pregnancy. Although you can't control how they respond to your invitation, you may find that they need to be with you and your baby during this time. It could be that they want to touch mom's belly, to sing or tell stories to the baby, to read favorite books, and to be present during some of the events and experiences during this special time. They will also need memories and shared family time as they cope with this deep loss themselves and try to help and support you over time.

As you might imagine, there will be ups and downs in the weeks and months ahead. Depending upon the choices you make, you may be able to spend many happy hours and days that will become even more important down the road as you remember and heal. Allow the mixed emotions to come as they do. Each has a place in your heart and your journey. This is your baby's story. This is your family story. Embrace it and be as present as you can. When you find yourself in need of support or someone to talk with, check out the many national and regional resources that may offer you advice, comfort, and a sense of community. You may also have any number of fears that should be addressed with someone who can appropriately respond. Toni-Marie was brutally honest about her fears,

> Thoughts that keep me up at night: After the doctors told me the lethal news about my baby and that he will die, I had several nightmares associated with his dying and death. Since I certainly never had a baby die on me, a million thoughts went through my mind, all which kept me up at night and set me off into panic attacks. For example, when the baby dies . . . in utero, Will I feel it? Will I know when it happens? Will I feel him die? Will it hurt? Will I gush blood? Then I want to know how and where you bury a baby, especially

since we have never even thought about our own endings and what we would do.

These raw and honest questions are hard to ask just anyone. From our experience with many parents, asking a doctor or midwife for medical advice is the logical place to start. Additionally, well-informed bereaved parents can be helpful, especially if they have training and stories of others in their hip pockets. This is a perfect time when a care companion, Baby Loss Family Advisor/Loss Doula, or Palliative Care Team can be of assistance. They have been asked such questions by many people, and if they are bereaved parents, they might have more credibility with mothers, who like hearing it from other moms' lips.

FEARS

The following are but some of the many fears parents tell us they faced after learning the news and choosing to continue the pregnancy to its natural state.

How will we look at this in years to come? Did we make the right decision for our baby and our family? A conversation worth having as often as you need. You are not alone in wondering this.

> Throughout my pregnancy and after Hazel's birth, the thing that was always on my mind when we had to make decisions was: "How will we feel about this in years to come, how will we live with this decision?" This was the foundation that I fell back on to try and enable us to come out the other side one day and be okay. —Vanessa, *Holding On & Letting Go: Facing an Unexpected Diagnosis in Pregnancy*

What will others think? Will they be talking behind my back and will it impact our family and even my work environment? Most parents express this concern and it is warranted. People do talk, and they do want to understand. Not because they want to hurt you, but rather because they are human, they care, and they need to talk through this to figure out how to best understand and support you. Usually they don't know what to do or say, so you, or some of your team, may need to let them know how to help (letters, e-mail, phone calls, or in-person visits with specific information that you want them to know and a few ideas about your immediate needs, such as nonjudgmental support, meals, help with housework or the children, time off work, etc.).

How do I begin to tell our other children and how shall we include them? This is discussed in chapter 20, "Supporting Your Children."

Will it hurt when the baby dies? Will I know? What do I do? Some mothers know approximately when their baby died and others do not. Rarely do they report pain. More often it is a feeling that something has changed, the baby is moving less, though not all moms feel this.

Will my pregnancy, labor, and birth now be handled differently at appointments and at the hospital during labor and delivery? Will they see me as a freak? An understandable fear felt by many. Talk with your medical provider about how things will proceed. Know that you are not the only one they have seen in this situation and they understand that this should be a happier time. Staff are concerned for you and will not blame you, and they should not treat you differently, except as is needed for your medical and emotional situation. Remember, many of them have been through this before with others.

Will I ever be able to smile or laugh again? Will this ruin my life and my happiness? It may feel like that now. But it won't forever. You will never "get over" this and will always remember your child and this time, but the details fade and the love for your baby and each other will glow brightly in time.

TIME WITH YOUR BABY

You should be given a chance—and encouraged—to meet your baby, if he dies prior to or at birth. It is possible that your baby will live for a while, so you'll need to think about how much intervention you want. The hospital team may have standards or protocols that they follow regarding how much they can or will do to intervene with a baby who has the problems your child has. If you are not happy with their suggestions or plans, ask to speak with someone else. Find out which department works with patients regarding rights and disputes about staff decisions. Given that your child's life may be short, the more you can discover prior to birth, the better. You don't want to be fighting a battle while parenting your precious bundle.

You will want to decide how much involvement you want with your child from the beginning. If you seek a high degree of time and care to give to your child, don't be surprised if some members of the hospital staff question you. They may honestly believe that the best way for you to cope is to not bond too much or to spend too much time with your baby. This is not their call and it is not helpful. Whether you realize it or not, you *have* bonded with your baby, and you may now realize that this is your time together. So stay strong and ask for help from family or an advocate and go up the chain of command if necessary. Thankfully, our experience has been that most hospital staff, especially neonatal intensive care unit (NICU) nurses and social workers understand the importance of spending quality time with your baby. They recognize that these are your rights and that this memorable time will serve you well over the long haul.

> When I learned that my niece's baby was in the NICU and would likely die soon, I immediately went to visit. I asked where my niece was only to have a nurse say, "I encouraged her to go home. Since the baby will die, it is better for her to not see her baby or spend time with her. That will only hurt her more. Better she forget and move on as soon as possible." I was shocked! Appalled! What kind of backward thinking coming from a NICU nurse who should have known better. Thankfully, Jenny came after I called and we met and held her baby for hours prior to his death. At least now she has no regrets and got to parent little Colton for a while. —An Auntie

PREPARATION

You may get help in crafting a birth vision/birth preferences plan (discussed in chapter 6, "Birth Plans and Preparation"), which can help you to maintain some sense of control as you prepare for the special labor and birth. It can also help your family and caregivers to know your wishes so that they can assist you in creating a beautiful hello and a memorable good-bye when that time comes (chapter 7, "The Labor and Birth"). Making the most of being involved parents to your child means being present and involved as fully as you are able to be in order to help you maximize your memories and minimize your regrets. If you follow this rather simple principle and know your intentions, you may find that other concerns can be dealt with in a relatively reasonable manner.

> My baby was carefully placed in my arms; I was in complete awe of how beautiful that little boy was. For a moment the world felt right. Time stopped, and the knowledge that he could soon be gone was forgotten. —Jennifer Ross, *Isaiah's Story*

You are courageous to follow your heart and let nature take its course. The time ahead is yet to be determined. There may be physical issues that arise, emotional struggles, and community and family pressures to deal with. This may also be the most meaningful time together with your baby that brings you joy and smiles. This is the time when your baby is safe within mom's womb and still a physical part of the family.

Don't be surprised if your feelings, fears, and doubts are intertwined with joy, happiness, love, and anticipation of meeting your baby. Though there will be sadness in knowing the ending before life outside the womb begins, you needn't let that define this important time with your child. That sadness is understandable and probably necessary, but keeping it in proper perspective to be dealt with later can be very helpful. You have this time and you won't get it back.

> We chose to put all the dark/tough feelings on hold, knowing they would be there waiting for us after our baby was buried and physically gone. The short time we had with Nathan needed to be honored and cherished. So that's what we did. Loved him up, talked with him, and experienced him fully. And we have no regrets. —Anonymous

Baby Items and the Baby's Room

This is one of the more difficult topics when you are pregnant with a baby who is likely to die. You may think that you don't need to buy anything for the baby or decorate a room, yet you may want to do so desperately. It is such an exciting and important parenting task that becomes another loss that adds to the heartbreak. You don't have to deprive yourself of all of the preparation and joy.

Although you may not know if your baby will get home or not (either alive or after death for a short time), you do have some choices and some options. You can still buy things for the baby, and you could do something to the baby's room in case she comes home. Of course, you know you will also have to make decisions about that room if or when the baby dies, but if it is something important that you want to do, do it. Don't allow the comments or concerns of others to influence you. As for the baby items, you can include them in the pictures you take of the baby after birth and you can give them as gifts to the baby's siblings or to other family members as mementos of your baby. You can even donate them to a local charity or save them to use for your next baby (if there is one). This is a sweet way to teach future siblings about their sibling who came before them.

If your baby does live for some time after birth and you get to bring her home, having a few items you made or purchased just for her can be very special.

> I am so happy we had both donated and purchased baby items in his room during the pregnancy. We did not expect Oliver to live, yet he did. For seventeen days. Having him in our bedroom, and occasionally in his own room, was really awesome. We dressed and undressed him, took lots of pictures in every room in the house, and had a birthday each and every day for him. We were able to unwrap presents each day that then became beautiful memories. Months after he died, we took those presents (toys and clothes) and gave them to our family and friends who were so supportive. Everyone got an Oliver present. Good thing we followed our instincts and got baby items and decorated his room a little during the pregnancy. We would never have left him with someone else in order to go buy things after his birth. —Anonymous

BONDING WITH YOUR UNBORN CHILD

You may have jumped in fully with every intention of staying positive and engaged during the entire pregnancy. Some parents can do this most of the time, and some ride the roller coaster up and down.

Given the situation, emotional withdrawals during the pregnancy can seem like a form of self-preservation. As parents, you may be protecting yourselves from all the emotions you may be feeling—such as grief, anger, sadness, and apprehension about a situation beyond your control—with short-lived escapes from your responsibilities and all the things that come with being pregnant. You may need a weekend away from home with your girlfriends. Or a visit to a spa might help. Respite will help reenergize you.

What usually comes naturally during typical pregnancies can take a lot of demanding work to keep going when carrying a child with a critical condition. You may be afraid that the heartbreak you are experiencing will be too much if you remind yourself and others of your pregnancy. Some parents are frightened that creating a bond with their baby will make the separation harder to bear. They believe that pulling away emotionally will lessen the pain in the short run. The opposite is probably true. Parental love cannot be controlled or limited. It is real and it is within you, no matter how much you try to believe it isn't there. It's true that when you love someone who is about to die, the pain is great for a long time. After all, that is a natural response to loving deeply. However, there can be much joy and love that shines through all that darkness, if allowed. We encourage you to welcome the hopes, dreams, and love, then embrace and enjoy your pregnancy as much as possible.

> My husband once said, "All that we can be sure of is *this* moment. Let's make the most of it." And so we did. We sang to them. We touched and caressed them through my tummy and my husband read *The Hobbit* story to them every night. —Nathalie Himmelrich, *Grieving Parents—Surviving Loss As a Couple*

There are several ways to bond with your unborn baby as you embrace pregnancy. We suggest you explore some of the following strategies and find the ones that suit you best.

Name Your Baby

When you give your unborn baby a name early, he or she becomes your son or daughter rather than a very sick fetus. A name helps make the baby a real part of your family and a sibling to your other children. Saying your baby's name aloud also invites others to talk about your child. However, if you are not ready to do this, don't. Some parents refer to their baby's nicknames: JLB (Jacob's little brother), Munchkin, or Sweet Pea. Think of what your intention is when you make this decision. Do you want to meet your child before giving a name? Do you fear that if you get too close and commit to a name it will hurt more? Or do you just feel that you are not yet ready for this step? In any case, you will figure out what you need to do.

> Saying his name out loud when alone was easy from the beginning. But saying his name in front of family took more courage at first. After awhile others spoke his name quite naturally. This helped us all. —A dad

Talk, Sing, or Play Music to Your Baby

From about sixteen weeks onward, your baby develops reactions to sound, recognizes your voice, and responds to different sounds. Music, family storytelling, and reading books and poetry are some ways to connect with your baby. Feel free to talk about anything, from cheerful subjects to the condition itself. The depth of your love will be communicated to your baby.

> I started to talk to my baby about her condition and explained to her what it meant in terms of consequences. It didn't feel funny to tell an unborn baby that she would die; I remember telling her that I would be there and had this overwhelming feeling that she already knew and understood the bigger plan. For me, talking about the unspoken was a way to accept, face, and forgive. —Stephanie

> When I found out Lana had spina bifida and a strong chance of having Down syndrome, I had to force myself to be maternal toward her. At the beginning, I was so ashamed and I ignored her and the pregnancy. After a while, I started talking to her, and as she moved more and more, we developed a quiet bond. By the time she was born, we were as close as I was to my older son. —Lana's mom

Massage Your Belly and Touch Your Baby

By touching your baby through your tummy, you are communicating with your baby. Many parents describe playing a gentle game of "kicking back," where they gently pushed the baby and the baby pushed back in return. Playing games with your baby can be a way of lightening the situation. Partners and children can also join in. Toward the end of your pregnancy, you may even be able to feel a bottom, a foot, or a head.

Follow Your Baby's Physical Development

When you follow your baby's progress, you will start visualizing him at different stages, giving him an identity. Find books, surf the Net, or download an app that shows the stages of the baby's growth. Take time to "see" your baby's growth. Don't forget to keep up with your prenatal care. It's just as important for you as it is for the baby. Continue your regular doctor's appointments and be good to your own body.

Involve Your Partner or Other Children

Involve your partner and any other children you have in the physical and emotional aspects of the pregnancy. Discuss the baby and what he or she has done each day (where you both went, if any noises startled her, when she got excited, if you played music for her). By involving others in your pregnancy, you may be giving others permission to talk about the baby and share your experience, both good and bad. This can bring you all together, offering sadness and joy at times, sharing fears and hopes, and giving each other support along the way.

> I've been pregnant before and knew how much attention the baby and I got. During this pregnancy, I missed family and friends asking about the baby, the pregnancy, and the process. In a way, it became another loss. Not only was I deprived of a healthy baby, but the silence we experienced during those many months was noticeable and oh so hard to bear. —A mom

Write to Your Baby

You may want to put your feelings down on paper. Whether in a journal, a letter, or simply on a notepad, tell your baby how you feel emotionally: your hopes, dreams, and realities; your thoughts about the diagnosis; and how you are coping as time goes on. Although this is highly emotional, it can release your emotions, helping you greatly in the grieving process.

CARING FOR YOURSELF

Exercise

Exercise can help to clear your mind and ease bodily tension. There are so many exercise options, including the simple act of daily walking or biking. While exercising, you can also enjoy your surroundings—sunset, sunrise, blooming trees, and flowers often bring a sense of peace. Try to clear your mind as you exercise, whether outside, in a gym, or in your own home. Not only is exercise useful for staying in shape and maintaining health, the endorphins that kick in as you exercise create a natural sense of wellbeing and even pleasure. Of course, before you embark on any exercise regimen, consult with your doctor.

Connect with Others

Networking and sharing your problems with friends can decrease stress levels. Some moms may feel like withdrawing from social scenes when they receive a prenatal diagnosis, however, receiving support can help. Connect with others and allow them to connect with you. One study found that women may not use the flight-or-fight method of coping with a crisis as much as men. Rather, they "tend and befriend," which may result from the additional oxytocin released by the brain. Thus, there may be a natural, physical response of needing to be around others as a way of coping.

Take a Daily Break

Take time each day exclusively for yourself, even just fifteen minutes. As a mom, you may have many responsibilities along with the emotional strain you are bearing. Stay strong and healthy; find the right balance. You might need to drop some activities to avoid becoming overwhelmed. Then focus on the ones that matter the most.

Seek Laughter

A good laugh by yourself or with someone else—whether while watching a comedy, reading a funny magazine, playing games, or telling jokes—can also help you unwind. Humor is the best medicine, so they say, and this may actually be true! Find opportunities to feel happy and to allow healthy distractions to entertain you for a moment here and there.

Pamper Yourself

Visit the hairdresser or go to a spa to help rejuvenate yourself. Pregnancy massages and manicures can be a nice time out. A bubble bath with soft music and candlelight is something free and easy to do. If you have child care issues, perhaps you can have someone take the children for an hour or two while you make time to bathe or pamper yourself. You deserve it and need it during the pregnancy.

Get Creative

If you are crafty, musical, or artistic, make some time to be in that creative space. According to Dr. Ivy Margulies, this type of outlet uses another part of your brain, which can provide a break and bring some peace and joy. Some moms described their pregnancies as triggers for change. They explained that they wanted to start something that they would do for a long time in memory of their baby or even just for a break. One mother began playing the piano, another redesigned her gardens, and others took up such activities as painting, knitting, needlepoint, or even woodworking. Still others volunteered for a charity, giving their babies a chance to be present while giving to others.

Inspirational Outlets

Many parents may feel intimidated about speaking their thoughts and feelings aloud, while others find it to be an easy and fulfilling means of expression. Writing can be cathartic and can include letters, journal entries, poetry, stories, and blogs. It is lasting and can be used to help others to understand what you are going through. Reading inspirational writings such as poetry, blogs, and books by other parents who have had this type of experience can be cathartic.

Restful Surroundings

Find surroundings that provide you with peace and a place to process your thoughts and emotions and even that give you space to create plans for your baby. Being in nature can be a natural relaxant. A lake, beach, meadow, forest, mountaintop, or valley may be just the place for you to think or escape. Whatever your preference, make time to seek and enjoy some restful spots where you can take a breather and relax.

> I found that being outside a lot made me feel better. I planted a lot of wild flowers and tended the roses every day. It made me feel better to see something growing and blossoming. —Anonymous

Change Your Surroundings

This might be the time for some small changes in your home. A distraction or change may be good for you. You could redecorate your house, paint some walls, rearrange furniture, or get new plants, curtains, or carpeting. Ask yourself what will bring positive energy into your space. If, however, you feel that any change is painful or threatens your safe, secure home, then keep things as they are. You will know what works for you. Changes may even include the lighting in the house, the tidiness, music, scents, and the general appearance.

Meditate or Use Guided Visualization

The purpose of meditation and guided visualization is to associate peaceful images with elevating thoughts in order to feel relaxed and less stressed. Though not for everyone, many moms find meditation and guided visualization quite useful. Meditation is the art of focusing your attention on an object, thought, or sound while breathing deeply. It can bring calm and positive thoughts. Visualizing images such as ocean waves, a meadow, a peaceful color, or clouds, for example, can also relax and calm.

I did relax while carrying Christopher. I sang to him, thought about him, and sent loving thoughts and energy to him. I think that is part of the reason he hung on for so long. The doctors truly thought it was a miracle that he lasted six weeks longer than they thought he would.
—Anonymous

Prayer and Spirituality

Many people instinctively pray or reflect on their lives and purpose when they experience trials, even if they hadn't used prayer much in their lives previously. Tragedies such as a death usually challenge people to reflect on a higher being, which can then encourage prayer.

Like many parents, you may find your faith in God deepens after your baby dies. Maybe you realize that you cannot face the loss alone. There are some parents who seem to find peace easier than others. They may even believe that their child is too pure or special for this earth. Many others rail against the tragedy and cry out, asking why their child has to die.

Aromatherapy

Occasional use of oils and scents in the air or on your skin may help you to relax. This can be done with a diffuser or scent sticks in the room or you can put the oil on your clothes (some can be used on your skin). You may even consider using of aromatherapy while in labor or at the hospital. However, you should do some homework on the Internet in case there are any side effects during pregnancy or labor.

Healthy Nutrition

Although it may seem odd to eat healthy foods when you know your baby will die, it still may make some sense to you. Perhaps you want to give your baby every chance you can. Also remember that you need to stay healthy, too. Feeling good about your part in this pregnancy is important, so do what feels right. There is also more to it than what foods you eat. For many people, meals are a means of socializing, a way to connect with friends and family. They are another way to find comfort and support. Enjoy some foods with people you love.

Breathing Exercises

Breathing exercises are the simplest and most straightforward techniques for relaxing. When you breathe deeply, you expand your lungs. Much of your good health involves your lungs. Take slow, deep breaths through the nose (say, for example, for four counts) and breathe out slowly through the mouth (twice as long—eight counts in this example). Do this regularly whether you are pregnant or not. Breathing helps with grief symptoms, anxiety, and overall well-being.

Physical Relaxation

While breathing deeply, you can also work on relaxing your whole body. Find a comfortable position, then begin at your feet tensing your muscles for a few seconds then releasing. Follow up to your legs, thighs, abdomen, back, shoulders and neck, then head. All the while, do your deep breathing in through the nose and out through the mouth. It may also help to focus on optimistic and positive thoughts.

Yoga

Yoga classes are often available in community or fitness centers. Although pregnancy yoga is tailored for you at the moment, consider the emotional impact of doing pregnancy yoga with other pregnant moms. Only you will know if this is something that you would like or whether you would prefer a mainstream yoga class. Yoga is a spiritual technique that helps to unite body and mind, and for some may even involve uniting with a higher being. Yoga exercises involve deep breathing and certain body positions. One goal of yoga is to find a balance between body and mind.

Acupuncture

Acupuncture is an ancient Eastern medicine technique that uses small needles inserted at acupuncture points in the skin. It is meant to help specific organs of the body and open up the body's chi. Acupuncture should only be performed by trained professionals. If you have doubts or concerns, check with your doctor or local professional association.

Hypnosis

Some people find hypnosis to be helpful with their issues and for making changes in their behaviors. Only trained hypnotherapists should perform hypnosis.

2

PALLIATIVE CARE AND PERINATAL HOSPICE

Now that you are committed to care for your baby through the pregnancy, you will probably seek experienced people and programs that can offer you tender care, wisdom, stories of others, and bonding opportunities during pregnancy, labor, and birth. If your family is new to this and you have never had such an experience, you may appreciate a navigator or guide. There are people who can aid you during your pregnancy and after the baby has been born. This type of care, called palliative care or perinatal hospice, is growing and has its origin in the hospice movement.

WHAT IS PERINATAL HOSPICE AND PALLIATIVE CARE?

Perinatal hospice and palliative care are interchangeable terms for a program of care that is instituted at many—though far from all—hospitals and also within communities. Its purpose is to help families carry babies with fatal or life-limiting diagnoses to birth and beyond. These programs also offer support after the baby is born or when she dies. Compassionate support, guidance, information, and resources are shared to ease the journey and support the families' wishes. This care paradigm is relatively new. A few doctors and key parents, including bereaved mother and pioneer Amy Kuebelbeck, along with her former nurse and colleague Annette Klein, have nurtured this movement. In a letter to honor her son Gabriel's fifteenth birthday and to thank those involved in promoting and delivering perinatal hospice care, Amy wrote of its history and present successes. She credits Dr. Byron Calhoun with starting the movement; he proposed and promoted the idea of perinatal hospice through articles in medical literature around 1999. When Amy discovered the practice and realized that there was a name for the type of care she and her husband sought for their son, she became a passionate champion. Prior to this there were so few resources to support parents who chose to continue, rather than end, their pregnancies. This lack of counsel and guidance resulted in a small number of parents choosing to continue their pregnancies.

Palliative care and guidance can begin at the time of diagnosis and continue until the time of death and beyond. The care itself is typically not in a hospice center but is provided to parents through in-person conversations, phone calls, e-mails, or even in groups. When the baby is born, help may be given in the hospital or at home once the baby is stabilized following birth (medical care is not usually provided at home, though a home health nurse may visit; ask about this if you are interested). This growing movement provides not only guidance, but can help you to increase your confidence in making your decision to continue with your pregnancy. The multidisciplinary care team may include doctors, nurses, genetic counselors, social workers, and chaplains, as well as experienced, trained parents. They work to empower you to be *active parents* to your child who will eventually die or may be born with special needs that might result in death at some point down the road. Fear lessens with such strong support. Confidence increases with the knowledge that there are people to turn to when questions and concerns arise.

On the website of Sufficient Grace, a ministry to help families facing this situation, perinatal hospice is referred to as "hospice in the womb," which includes birth planning and support after baby's birth until death and beyond. They write, "We want parents to know they are not walking this path alone."

There are many issues covered under the perinatal hospice program. Pain management and plans for labor and birth are a few. Personal care decisions for mom and baby, memory making, and planning a meaningful good-bye are other services that can be provided, along with bringing baby home and all that goes with that. Preparing for the unexpected is addressed, since each birth and baby are unique and often involve unexpected changes that can't be controlled or planned for. Since there are so many options to be considered, the medical staff may or may not be prepared for such in-depth discussions unless they have perinatal hospice program and training or are certified Loss Doulas or Baby Loss Advisors. Although perinatal hospice programs are becoming more prevalent in some communities, you will need to determine whether your professionals are trained and engaged in such deep, passionate care practices.

HOW DOES IT WORK?

Support people are invited by the staff, with parent permission, to directly contact parents. They either call or e-mail to offer help. If a meeting is possible, that is set up. But if not possible due to distance or scheduling issues, conversations occur via phone or e-mail. The advisor or hospice worker listens to the parents' concerns and offers thoughts on options for how to proceed. He or she shares other parents' stories and gives permission to the parents to create their own journey. The advisor/hospice worker then helps the parents to begin doing some birth visioning to help create a birth plan for the rest of the pregnancy, for the actual birth, and for meeting baby. The parents and circumstances usually determine the timing and speed. The advisor/hospice worker also shares information with parents about the consequences of their choices, along with many resources.

The parent support people at this time may be referred to as advocates, navigators, care companions, nurse navigators, Baby Loss Doulas, Baby Loss Family Advisors, or palliative or hospice volunteers. For a list of independent, caring advisors, visit www.BabyLossFamilyAdvisors.org or www.StarLegacyFoundation.org for care companions. Even if none are physically located in your community, they can help you by phone or e-mail. This is common and the feedback has been positive.

Sherokee acted as a Loss Advisor and helped Toni-Marie, whose son was destined to die later in her pregnancy. Toni-Marie e-mailed that she was worried about going to her sister's wedding because no one in her family knew that her baby would die prior to or shortly after birth.

She wanted to be happy for her sister, but was upset and sad about her baby.

After Sherokee e-mailed her affirming messages and specific suggestions, Toni-Marie wrote,

> Your words for the wedding were exactly what I needed to hear. You are right. This will be his first wedding, and wedding ceremonies are so loving and the surroundings will be beautiful and peaceful. Plus, because I am *in* my sister's wedding, that means so will the baby. Any picture I take means he will be with me. You just made me realize how special that is going to be. He will be there with me as I'm with her and my other family. Her wedding pictures will be pictures of his only life and I am realizing I will cherish this forever. Thank you for that. Seriously, thank you for making that point.

Later she wrote, "You are like my personal journal. You let me vent my feelings and 'crazies' and then teach me how to go forward with choices and resources. I couldn't go forward during this very, very difficult time without your calm, reassuring guidance."

This is the kind of conversation that can be had with someone who understands what you are going through and can provide you with alternative perspectives. Look within your community or on the Internet for legitimate groups that provide these types of support people.

HOSPITAL OR COMMUNITY PROGRAMS

If your hospital is not familiar with it or does not have a program, call the nearest hospice program and ask about perinatal hospice, since it is becoming an integral part of hospice programs. You deserve this tender and well-informed care, but if your local hospital does not yet fully understand the importance or for another reason has not implemented a perinatal hospice program, you will need to seek help from others. As a backup option if there are no local experts, you may wish to look other places to find care providers who can help you immediately. Visit the website www.perinatalhospice.org to find lists of programs available throughout the world, as well as studies, articles, and other resources. You may also wish to invite a birth planner, Baby Loss Family Advisor or Baby Loss Doula (www.LossAdvisors.org), or a locally trained care companion to assist you in preparing for what is ahead. These professionals will be knowledgeable about many of your options and can assist with birth planning, offer listening ear during the journey, and may even be assist you at or after the birth.

TIPS AND ADVICE

- The first place to look for a list of palliative care programs is the website www.PerinatalHospice.org. There you will find hundreds of programs throughout the United States and the world. Clearly, not all available programs are listed there, so don't use it as your only source, but it may provide an area program that is easy to locate.
- If you didn't find one listed near you, contact your local hospitals and ask someone to help you locate a perinatal hospice or palliative care program. You can start by calling the maternal nurse manager or administration. Learn who the director or coordinator is and get in touch. Ask questions about how it works and if you can get help soon. It is usually free of charge, but if you are wondering, do ask. If the hospital does not have such a program and cannot help you to find one, look up area hospice programs and explain your situation. Ask for help in preparing for a gentle, planned birth and time with your baby if she survives.
- Make a list of questions and concerns you may have, such as having more or less care than the doctors recommend. Since this is your baby, you would think you would have full say. This is not always what happens, however.

> Our baby had hypoplastic left heart syndrome, which meant he would be in for a lifetime of surgeries, medication, or a heart transplant, beginning immediately following birth. We could not imagine putting him through that much pain and distress, especially given that he may not live long anyway. When we told our doctor our plan to forgo all surgery and let the baby dictate his own life play, we were shocked at the response. They went so far as to threaten taking it to the hospital board to force us to have the surgeries. Thankfully we found a sympathetic perinatal loss specialist who recommended we find another doctor who would honor our wishes. We did that. Our son lived less than a week, but he

went on his terms and we were with him every minute. No regrets. —A mom

Create a birth plan as early as you can; feel free to revise it as you
learn more and explore your options further. You may want to have
someone assist you as you create it or look it over when you're finished to help ensure you have covered all your bases. If your hospital
does not have an expert to help with this (most palliative care programs have people who know how to do this), use our resource section at the end of this book to find online or telephone support from
care companions and advisors. You may even find someone in your
local area or get a referral from someone on this list.

- Share some or all of your birth plan with your family and close
friends so that they know what to expect. This may also give them
ideas about how to help. For example, if you say you want a homelike
service or celebration, someone may offer to coordinate the food or
even offer a venue if you can't have it in your own home.
- Ask your family outright how they might wish to contribute. You may
not realize or remember their skills and talents.

> We didn't think to ask our parents what role they wanted to play.
> Once the service was over, we had a heartfelt conversation and
> learned that my father-in-law had wished he could have built the
> baby's casket (he is a master carpenter) and my mother wished
> she could have coordinated the food and made our daughter's
> dress and blanket. How special would that have been! Why didn't
> we ask? Why did I learn this so late? —Anonymous

If your plans change, go forward with the new ones. Don't feel
wedded to your initial plans. Communicate the change to your family, especially those who will be intimately involved.

- Talk to your baby. Explain what will probably happen. Share your
wishes and dreams along with your sadness. Voicing it may make you
feel better, and perhaps your baby will receive the message of love
you are sending.
- Check in occasionally with your palliative care contact. Clarify if she
or he will be an advocate for you when needed. Share changes in the
plan and ask questions that concern you. Feel the love and support of
the palliative care team. They are there for you.

- If you wish to talk with other mothers or fathers who have been down this road, ask for contacts. Some parents report that it is difficult to reach out to a stranger, so don't worry if this is also difficult for you. A better approach is to suggest that these parents contact you. If they happen to call at a bad time, you can call back when you are free. Be sure to get their number so you can call back.
- Honesty is best, though not always easy. If you are worried about how your child will look, how to tell your other children, if you will feel pain if the baby dies prior to birth, or what to do to minimize awkwardness when you return to work, just put it out there. No question is a dumb one. Remember, you have never been through this before, how can you know *any* of the answers?
- If you want to bring your baby home, talk with your provider about whether and how this could be done. If you want to have your baby at home to live and die, whenever that time comes, talk with your provider. It may be that you'll need to get some medical equipment to assist or that there may be other complications. But don't give up trying unless you come to an impasse. You never know what is possible. Since you don't get another chance at this, think big. If it is hard for you to do this type of negotiation, take an advocate with you to the table for this conversation. And be sure someone takes good notes.
- After your baby is born and when you have some time, fill out any evaluations you were given or write a note to the hospital team. Tell them what helped you and what you wish could have been different. They need this feedback to improve their program, and it may feel good to put what happened and your feelings on paper.

> Following Brennan's death, I felt so alone and empty. What now? I wondered. Then I remembered I had been given an evaluation of the birth and care. For the next few hours, I practically wrote a book. I shared the good things we appreciated, what my labor was like, and who did what and how it helped. Later, after thinking about things, I also wrote a letter to the hospital about what hurt us and what I wish should be changed. Those suggestions were read. I received a call soon after, inviting me to speak to the doctors and nurses about how to improve care for families like ours. I am so grateful I communicated and that they really listened and even wanted more. —Sherokee

3

PRESSURE FROM OTHERS TO CHANGE YOUR MIND

You made a decision and want others to respect that. However, parents-to-be report receiving pressure to end abnormal pregnancies from medical professionals and even family members. You may have felt pressure soon after you shared the news, or you may have heard it after making your decision. It may occur because carrying an unhealthy baby to term seems unusual. In past decades many parents-to-be felt that their only choice was to end the pregnancy. Continuing the pregnancy and accepting the outcome—no matter the severity—has not been as common and was rarely discussed. Since others probably cannot imagine knowingly going through a pregnancy, only to have the baby die or be severely disabled, you may be questioned often about this decision. Medical professionals may also worry about your emotional and psychological well-being during this time and suggest ending a pregnancy so that you do not have to endure all that goes with the choice you made.

PROTECTING YOU

These well-intentioned people don't want to see you hurt; they are trying to protect you. Doctors and loving family members may also be unable to support you well because it is uncomfortable and painful for *them*. What can they possibly do or say to make this any easier? Doctors are trained to save lives, not to give care to mothers-to-be who know their babies may die but want to continue the pregnancy anyway. If they can't save the baby, they wonder why parents would choose to go forward in this way. And if you move on quickly, you can get pregnant again sooner. Although not all doctors feel this way, many do, so don't be surprised if you encounter them. Family members may have similar philosophies. Their tears and fears for you, your baby, and for themselves compound the confusion about what to say. Privately, they may wonder why you would put yourself through this type of torture.

FEELING UNDERMINED

Consequently, you may receive messages that undermine your decision. Even if they don't say it aloud, you may feel judgment or concern. They are not trying to hurt you; rather, it is their way of being supportive. They may also think this is better for you and the baby. They don't know and probably can't love this baby as her parents can. So they may not understand the depths of your despair at the thought of your baby dying as a result of termination. And they surely may not understand either how you could want to prolong that death for months as you carry and nurture your child or how you could live with a challenged child for the rest of her life.

Given these reasons, it may not surprise you to know that a number of mothers report that at subsequent clinic visits they were asked repeatedly to reconsider. The subject of pregnancy termination continued to come up. Doctors and even some genetic counselors questioned if the right decision had been made; they worried about mothers' stress. You will go through months of appointments with a challenged pregnancy only to birth a baby who will not live or live well. This is not easy for them, and they probably have little experience with it. When they continually challenge your decision, it can feel like you have to repeat the steps that got you there. It may also feel like they are undermining you.

One couple commented about their frustration with caregivers who did not support their decision or who continually undermined them. In *Giant Hero*, Cecil reported, "He then told us 'You mean you are to *keep* this baby?' I said, 'You are darn right! That's our baby. . . . We are not going to give up on him.'" Another couple commented, "We were shocked that the genetic counselor kept repeating 'incompatible with life.' It upset us both deeply. Why did it matter to her? We had already decided to keep the baby and let nature take its course. Clearly, she didn't get it and we weren't going to change her mind."

> She was listed as incompatible with life and we were advised by our medical care provider to avoid her several times. We decided to keep her and let God take us wherever we were to go with this baby. —Andy B.

Since more couples and single moms are continuing their pregnancies, there may be more support for this decision. But if you do experience pressure or continued questions about your decision to carry the baby, you will need to be assertive and strong. Tell these people that you don't find their messages helpful, and in fact they are hurtful. Send a letter asking for their support. Tell them your mind is made up and that you need their support. You could even ask them not to bring up the subject up again. Tell them that your decision is final; you have your reasons and you ask them to support you, not to plant seeds of doubt. It is difficult enough to be on this path; you will want to be cared for and surrounded by people who trust your judgment and who will help you, not second-guess you. If your doctor does not follow your wishes and it is becoming stressful, you may need to look for another care provider.

> We thought getting the news that our baby was seriously ill and would likely die was the hardest thing. Deciding to care for him until he died, either in utero or shortly after birth, was the choice we made, though we weren't sure we knew how to actually do that. But what happened next made things even worse—our genetic counselor and doctor asked us if we were certain about this decision at every appointment and even when we called with questions or got test results back. It was horrible. With each conversation, we felt we were challenged to rethink the decision. Our anger grew to the point where we had to find different providers. Parents need support, not to be continually harassed. —A mom and dad

> Our providers were so very supportive. They gave us a book on decision making, talked it through with us, shared appropriate resources, and even hooked us up with other parents who had also continued the pregnancy. We felt so loved and supported. No one

questioned our decision once it was made. We were blessed.
—Nancy

TIPS AND ADVICE

- Examine your decision. How final is it? If you are committed, then be prepared to draw a line in the sand if need be.
- When you hear medical professionals begin to go down the road of questioning or appearing to judge your decision, kindly and firmly stop them and suggest that you have already made your choice. No going back, no need to revisit the issue.
- Maybe you can talk with a social worker or nurse and lay out your strategy for going forward, which includes not rehashing the past. Tell him or her that you need the support of your care providers and don't appreciate any pressure to take a different path.
- If you don't get anywhere with your care provider, start looking for another, if that is an option.
- If that is not an option, then take someone with you to appointments who can be your voice when you are pressured. Explain that you won't be second-guessed. Your energy is needed to do the hard work of living through the pregnancy and birth of your baby. Even more energy and strength will be needed to survive what happens after that.
- If you have a supportive caregiver who doesn't question your decision but gives you great support, thank him or her. Consider sending a complimentary letter to him or her and to the administration of the facility. All too often they receive only letters of criticism. If you appreciate the care, let them know, so they can feel good about continuing to offer this type of support to others.
- Some parents have reported that they were deeply upset by their doctors or genetic counselors who would not stop the pressure tactics. After the pregnancy was over, so as to avoid stirring up more tension while trying to enjoy and be with their baby, they wrote a letter either to the care provider or to their board complaining about the problem. Some considered it a formal complaint. If this is something you must do, then do it when you are ready and have the

energy for that battle. People can change and feedback or complaints can bring about change.

- It may be even more difficult to deal with family members who are pressuring you to reconsider your decision, since you are emotionally involved with them for the long term. Be honest and tell them face-to-face if you can. If that seems hard to do, write them letters or ask one of your advocates to communicate your message. Be kind, but firm. You have a right to follow your heart and to do what you need to do.

- Since family and friends may be acting out of fear that they don't know how to support you during this unusual time, let them know what you need. Be specific. You can say, "What would really help are words of encouragement about the pregnancy. Ask how it is going, if the baby moves much, if I have purchased baby items, and even where I have taken the baby." Tell them not to think about the outcome, but rather about the love you all have for this baby. Ask them to treat this pregnancy as normal as possible; this is the time you have with your baby, who is still safe within mom. You don't want it ruined by negativity or worry. Having a clear idea about what you specifically want may help other family members to be more willing to offer it to you.

- There will be some (medical professionals, family, or friends) who just can't get to where you are. They do not understand and may never. That is *their* problem, not yours. Don't let it alter your course, and don't give it much thought. You don't live in their minds and bodies; you live in yours. Work to forgive them and to move forward. Give them grace to disagree with you. If ever they find themselves in a similar situation, they will do it their way and you may not agree. But this is *your* life.

4

FAMILY DYNAMICS

DEALING WITH OTHERS

Interacting with others in the early days following your decision can be stressful. Some know what has happened, but most probably do not. Your energy may be focused on your nuclear family now, yet other people are waiting anxiously in the wings, many who are ready and waiting to be asked for help.

You will likely have needs in the days and weeks ahead. Even when it's difficult, be forthright. You can ask someone to do research for you. For example, maybe you'll want to know how to meet your baby; where to buy special gowns or blankets; where to find a beautiful small wooden casket; what the hospital rules and state and local laws are regarding bringing your baby home to die or after death; or what it's like to have a baby in the neonatal intensive care unit, including your rights such as holding your baby and how to give your baby your milk, even if breast feeding is not an option. This is a way to include family and friends. You may find that they will be more supportive in the future if they are included in the early days after the diagnosis and during the early days of your pregnancy.

Feel free to share your pregnancy news along the way with those who are supportive. You can share the times when your baby moves and your state of mind, along with other pregnancy symptoms. You are a mom who is still pregnant and who has the same experiences and concerns. If you can talk about it, share your plans for the pregnancy, for the birth, and for when or if your baby dies. For example, if you have decided to have balloons, pink or blue flowers, or other special ceremonies and mementos, let others know. Maybe they can help you with some of those things, which gives them a role and a way to offer you support. They are at a loss about how to help; invite them to get involved and give them jobs. This is a way of sharing a small part of your child's story with friends and family. The more you bring them into the loop, the more involved they will likely be later.

If your baby is likely to live but have health challenges, you can still share what you are learning and what you want during the birth and beyond. Maybe you would like help researching how to care for a special needs child. Remember, whatever the disability, your child is a precious individual with his or her own potential and uniqueness. Do not (and do not let others) underestimate the special life your child will live and the potential emotional gifts you will receive.

How to Answer Questions

Prepare answers for the questions of friends and strangers who inquire about your pregnancy or your baby. Since you are visibly pregnant, others will notice when you are in public. What used to be joyful questions from friends and strangers now may be painful and difficult to handle. Even if you tell everyone in your family and your close friends, there will be others who feel compelled to touch your growing belly and to ask about your baby. Pregnancy is such a special event that they probably can't help themselves. And they don't know your story.

You have a choice about whether and how you answer. You may change the subject, though be aware that they may bring the conversation right back to your pregnancy or they may ask again another time. You can prepare yourself ahead of time so you are not caught off-guard. You could say, "There are problems with the baby and I prefer not to talk about them right now." Or you might say, "When and if you really want to know and have the time, I will fill you in about what is going on during a private conversation." It is acceptable not to share the full story with everyone; you don't owe them that. However, if your family and friends do understand the situation well enough, they may be able to be more supportive—that is, if this is their style of interaction. For awkward moments with strangers, you may opt to simply thank them for their kind wishes and move along.

Couple Communication

Here you are as a couple facing weeks or months of pregnancy with an unexpected ending. Getting to this place as a couple probably has been stressful, given the high emotions and seriousness of the decisions you have had to face. Such heartbreaking news is never expected. And now you have made a decision to go forward with the pregnancy, knowing that it will be far from easy, though hopefully it will hold some joy. Tension that arises in any number of situations can put a strain on relationships. When it relates to your beloved child, of course the anxiety is intense. No one prepared you for this.

Staying Together

Whether married or not, you are a couple in a relationship that needs to survive and that hopefully grows stronger despite the stress. You will need to continue talking and supporting one another throughout the pregnancy, the birth, meeting your baby, and possibly saying good-bye. There will be many more decisions and forks in the road during this time. Should you take the extra tests? Do you want to focus on the positive or the negative? How do you embrace and live through the pregnancy? What do you say to others? How do you keep showing your love to one another when under such stress? In what special ways will you meet your baby? There are no simple answers about how to decide these things together. However, there are some philosophies to follow. The short version is: keep talking, remember that you love one another, communicate continually with one another, show one another respect even if you disagree, and do your best to continue to be the parents of this baby who knows your love and will always be loved by you.

> All the world as I knew it stopped. Some part of me had to continue being a new mother: expressing milk and changing nappies; loving my daughter. At the same time I was saying good-bye to the child who would never grow up with her sister, never hold hands while walking along the side of the road, never play with each other side-by-side, and most of all, the pain of never experiencing the special

bond that only identical twins share, a connection that I had only heard and read about. A few months back, in a very dark moment of self-judgment and self-hatred I told my husband: "You have the luxury to choose whether you want to stay with me or not. I do not have that luxury. I am stuck with myself without the likelihood of ever becoming that person again that I once was!" —Nathalie Himmelrich, *Grieving Parents—Surviving Loss As a Couple*

You will experience feelings of loss throughout this time, knowing that the end may be coming or that raising a child with severe challenges is ahead. Loss and grief continues for a long time and will impact you during pregnancy. Don't be afraid of it, and don't let it overwhelm you as you try to enjoy this special family time that will be all too short. Be slow to draw lines in the sand about what you will and will not do. It is only later, when you look back, that you may wish that you had been more willing to embrace the baby or that you may be better able to understand one another's requests and needs. Even if you are uncomfortable about some things, stay open and think about how you might look at this months or years after your baby has died. You get no "doovers." All the time you have together is now and the limited time you get with your child after birth.

Going out in public may be painful and awkward for both parents. How do you answer the questions about your pregnancy? "When is your baby due?" "Do you know the sex?" and so many other questions are no longer fun or even seem possible to answer. However, staying home also adds stress if you put your life on hold. Live your life and give your baby and one another time and attention now.

After your baby is born, there will be additional issues that arise. If your baby dies, you will experience grief and you will need to continue communicating and understanding one another. There is so much more you can do to keep your relationship strong and minimize the chance of losing one another. Read more about this in chapter 18, "How Men and Women Grieve and Get Along," especially noting the resources for couples.

Singles

Being a single mom who chose to continue an uncertain pregnancy is not where you expected to be. Whether you had an active partner who has left or is not present for some reason or if you never really had a partner when you got pregnant, you will need to find faithful support from others to help you through this. Even if you wanted to do it alone, consider reaching out for help. A typical pregnancy is a strain on any woman, and your pregnancy will be far from typical.

There will be people who tell you to be grateful that your baby will die, since parenthood will tie you down. Misunderstandings and hurtful comments add to your pain. Don't take them too seriously.

> Being young and single has not helped me get support. I hear too many comments about how I am fortunate not to have a (live) baby in my future. Now I can finish college and get a good job, they say. As if that will solve my sadness and fix me. The whole thing sucks. Why can't people just help me where I am? A mom whose baby will die. Period! I need support, not this. —A young mom

You may find (or could create) a Facebook group for other singles who are facing challenges in their pregnancies. You can be sure they are out there; there just aren't as many. Being with friends who are expectant couples during this time can be helpful, especially if they have had a similar experience. To them, helping you can be very therapeutic and special. A counselor can also help you during this tough time. Read chapter 19, "Single Moms," for more information.

5

MEDICAL ISSUES

As a parent who has a growing baby who will likely have medical issues, you may be worried and full of questions. Along with doing research and spending time as a family with your baby during this pregnancy, you may also be swamped with medical appointments, tests, and challenges different from those of a woman with a typical pregnancy. Do what you can to normalize your pregnancy and think about how to live through it in the best way that you can.

GATHERING INFORMATION

Hopefully, you have good relationships with your doctors, who encourage you to call or go to the office whenever you feel the need. You will have many questions, and issues will come up for which you are not prepared. Be sure that you know who to call and where to go when the unforeseen happens. Although collecting information on the Internet can be very informative and helpful, it can also provide false or confusing information. You'll want to keep a list of those kinds of topics to discuss with your doctors. If you find pictures and outcomes to be depressing and upsetting, that may be a clue to stop looking. You are already under enough stress; perhaps you should limit the kinds of information that puts additional stress on you and causes even more fear and confusion. This is your baby, not someone else's. You will see your own baby through your loving parental eyes. And she will probably look perfect to you.

On the other hand, search for and gather this information if you don't feel upset or stressed by it. Follow your heart and your head. Just remember, some of the stories and information you find may not be truthful or helpful.

> When my husband and I first learned that John Carl was going to die, I immediately Googled the medical terms to gather as much information as I possibly could to learn everything about the conditions, including looking at pictures, which were some of the most horrible images of dead babies who had similar diseases. I would stare at these pictures crying for days. But when I would ask my husband if he wanted to look, too, he would refuse. At first I was upset because, [why was he] not coping the way I was by spending hours on the Internet looking this stuff up and staring at the photos of these dead babies? But he explained to me that he was not interested in looking at other people's babies. He told me our baby is our baby and any picture I may be staring at on the Internet is not our sweet baby boy but someone else's. Those were not pictures of his baby and he had no interest in comparing. He said because our baby has yet to be born, he simply prefers to save that space in his brain so when the times comes he will make his own mental memories.
> —Toni-Marie

THE DEVELOPMENT OF YOUR PREGNANCY

There are already many books about pregnancy and what to expect. You probably have some of those books on your bookshelves already. Many parents expecting a child with a medical condition find that reading such books and websites about "normal" pregnancies and happy, healthy babies is difficult.

We are unaware of any book about the medical and emotional aspects of pregnancy that is written specifically for each abnormality that might be diagnosed. This is not something that we feel we can cover in this book. Therefore as you prepare for the rest of your pregnancy, you'll need to look beyond the painful or troubling information you find. Keep in mind that while diagnoses may be the same from pregnancy to pregnancy, the expression of those abnormalities may be different from child to child. Your baby may not look anything like another baby with the same diagnosis. There are also degrees of severity that might alter the way a delivery and life may go—some babies may die instantly while others live for hours, days, or weeks, even with the same fetal diagnosis. There are a number of resources at www.perinatalhospice.org. Hopefully, some of the resources and information can help you navigate medical and other pregnancy issues.

Of course, with an abnormal pregnancy, complications may arise. You should discuss the potential complications with your doctor. In some cases, you may deliver prior to your due date or you may require a special type of delivery. Knowing the medical procedures and outcomes you might expect will help you to better prepare. In addition, choosing a hospital for the special kind of care you and your child may need at delivery is important. Learning what a hospital will and will not do for an ill child may impact which hospital you choose for delivery.

It is essential to remember that your health is just as important as your baby's health. So don't neglect your own health during this difficult pregnancy. Make sure that you take any medications you're supposed to take and that you continue any routine medical exams such as eye appointments. Pay attention to any changes in your own health, and report them to your doctor.

Some things you may consider in the weeks and months ahead follow.

Baby Kicks

When you feel your baby move, you may have mixed feelings due to your diagnosis and decision. Prior to that, each kick and movement may have been exciting, a sign that the baby was "alive, healthy, and kicking." What you think about it and how you respond to it has now probably changed. You realize that you are carrying a baby who may only be with you for a short time or who may have a serious disability. Surely the love you feel for him does not change. However, now that you know that time with your child is limited, those movements are special reminders of a precious life.

At times, you may find yourself dwelling on what will happen in the future, what it will be like if she dies or needs much medical attention.

Instead of always preparing yourself for that painful future, work on being in the present. You can choose to view each movement as a gift. Your child is still alive and safe within mom. She should not be feeling any pain and she knows the love of her family. Maybe you can even take some video of the kicking that occurs near the end of pregnancy; this will be special in the years ahead.

You may have been told to take notice of your baby's movements in order to watch for signs of distress. If you are not sure what to do when this happens, talk with your medical provider. You may want everything possible done to help you have your baby alive in your arms, which might mean your provider has agreed to induce or schedule a caesarean. These are the types of decisions you will want to consider when you develop the birth plan or at medical appointments. If your doctor is not on the same page as you and this is causing you distress, you may want to interview other doctors. There may be someone in your area who is willing to help you try to have your baby while still she is still alive.

Changes with the Baby

Depending on your child's condition, some organs may not have formed or you may notice variations in your baby's development. Many babies are small for their gestational age, others may have larger heads, and some have fluid collecting around their organs. For instance, with Turner syndrome, the baby will probably be small, whereas a baby with Hydrops fetalis would be abnormally large due to fluid retention. Talk with a specialist about your baby's condition so you know what to expect. For instance, in cases where there is little amniotic fluid, the baby may be in breech position.

There have been stories of miraculous changes as the baby nears term, and problems that were viewed as incompatible with life lessened or disappeared. It is difficult to explain how problems (mostly nongenetic and probably less severe) clear up. Some describe them as miracles, while others suggest that since we have had the benefit of ultrasound's window into the womb for only a short period of time, some of these problems may occur and then go away or lessen naturally by the time the baby is near or at term. We don't want to get your hopes up, but it is appropriate to know that things may change during the pregnancy. With some disorders, the baby could improve or worsen. With no guarantees, you will need to remain flexible and vigilant. Also be sure to ask your doctor how the baby's health issues may impact your own. You'll need to take care of your body as well.

> We were told early in the pregnancy that there were some problems, including serious fluid collecting around our baby's organs and that it could be a lethal condition. It was suggested that we could end the pregnancy (or not). We decided to continue and asked for prayer constantly. A few days before birth, the miracle occurred. No more fluid. Even though the neonatal doctors were put on standby for the birth, our daughter came out screaming and healthy. We are ever grateful we did not end that pregnancy. —T & M

Impending Birth

As a pregnant mother, you may be feeling extremely tired and hypersensitive. Not only are you a mother ready to give birth, but you are experiencing the uncertainties and stress that usually accompanies a wanted pregnancy with a scary outcome. How do you deal with the emotional and mental anguish of preparing for the possibility of bringing a child with special needs home or organizing a funeral? And you may not be ready to let go of your precious child in your womb. Dad may be concerned about his role and frustrated by the unknown when the baby is born.

Keep communicating with your provider and family during this time. Have your bag packed early and remember to seek the information you need to help calm and prepare you.

TIPS AND ADVICE

- Make sure that you feel comfortable asking questions to your midwife, doctor, or social worker. Be honest and upfront about what you need to know and take time to process their answers.
- Ask your medical team about the services they offer. Will they refer you to counseling or psychosocial support? Can you have your ultrasounds and visits at the same location? How do they support women who have chosen to carry their pregnancies to term?

- Be careful where you seek your information. Many parents have had negative experiences searching for answers on the Internet, in magazines, or through hearsay. Be careful that what you find is relevant to your particular situation.
- Find yourself a good pregnancy companion book or app on your phone or tablet. Read about each developmental stage leading up to birth and watch your baby's progress as time goes on.

6

BIRTH PLANS AND PREPARATION

Your child's birth will forever remain a special day for you and your family. After his or her birth and whether she or he is born still, lives for a minutes or a year, ·your baby will remain your child forever.
—Anonymous

INCREASING CONTROL

Preparation for the impending birth of your baby is important whether you plan to take your baby home from the hospital or not. There are several things you can do to prepare yourself for labor and delivery. Writing down your plan can help you gain control. It can also help you deal with and overcome some of the fears. By working with someone experienced in helping parents like you develop a birth plan or birth vision, you will be led to topics and places you might not have imagined. And you will be grateful you went there when the time comes. Such preparation is also an important communication opportunity between you and your partner, if you have one. If not, you can designate a person close to you to join you in this discussion if you wish or you can do it by yourself. In the latter situation, it will be extremely helpful to have the assistance of a birth planning advisor. If your medical professionals do not offer you this service, refer to "Baby Loss Advisors" in "Resources" at the end of this book.

WHAT IS A BIRTH PLAN?

A birth plan is a written record of your wishes regarding labor, birth, family involvement, meeting your baby, ideas for memory making and good-byes, and more. As parents-to-be, there are reasons to create a specific, yet flexible birth plan or birth vision. Most parents find it helpful to think through the many choices available during labor, birth, and the time that follows with their baby—this is true whether the baby has already died, will die, or may live for some time with significant challenges. It takes into account your personal, spiritual, and cultural wishes when planning for the birth and its aftermath.

A birth plan can include such things as

- Preferred labor position
- Medication preferences
- Intervention strategies including any medical interventions
- Who will be in the delivery room
- Who will be in the waiting area
- What to bring to the hospital, including camera or video recorder
- Who will cut the cord (a great job for the father, who has so little to do during this important time)
- How you want to meet your baby if she is not immediately taken for care (this can include skin-to-skin contact with both parents; soothing music and smells; special blankets and clothing; memento creation; how and when to introduce her to siblings; and testing and autopsy decisions)
- Who will hold the baby after birth, especially if the baby will die soon
- Plans for taking the baby home, where he may die soon or live for some time
- Plans for family transport of the baby and for time at home if the baby has already died (if legal in your state or region)
- How to plan for and say your special good-byes, if baby dies

Depending upon your specific situation and your baby's problems, you may need to plan for contingencies—if the baby dies at or around birth and if the baby lives for some time. That may mean you will want to think about how to say your hellos and start your good-byes at the hospital, as well as making some plans for home care if your baby survives and you take him home for a short time.

Not everyone is ready to talk about planning for a child's death or impending life and death issues while still pregnant. If you are one, you certainly have permission to choose what to actively plan for. The questions and topics in the birth plan will at least stimulate thoughts and plant seeds for you, whether you actually complete one or not. Most parents who understand the purpose of birth planning eventually choose to do one and to find some help to ensure they do it well.

There are many parents who believe God can make miracles happen. They may believe that there is power in prayer and are hoping for a miracle. Therefore they wish to remain positive, avoiding the topic of death altogether. The main downside to this is that if the baby does die, the planning time is shortened. However, this can be overcome with good support and the use of practical resources. On very rare occasions, the predicted expectations for the baby's health are different than the outcomes. The medical community does not have a crystal ball when it comes to predicting exactly what will happen to babies during the rest of the pregnancy. Sometimes nongenetic issues clear up or are less dire than expected. Although we don't want to encourage you to hold out hope for one of those rare miracles or a better-than-expected outcome, we also don't want to burst your bubble if you are hopeful and need that hope to go forward. Therefore, your planning and preparing is a very personal process; trust yourself to make decisions that are right for you and your family.

The plan ought to be viewed as a flexible plan that serves as a general guide to help you and your caregivers while at the hospital. Inevitably, situations change during labor and delivery and what you thought would happen might not. Ideally, your birth plan is saved on your computer or even handwritten. A more casual option—a bulleted list or notes in a notebook—can also work; however, this leaves details to the interpretation of others. How you choose to do it may depend on the purpose. It can be as short or as extensive as you wish, in bullet-point format, essay format, or include both. If it is to serve primarily as a reminder to you during the chaotic hospital time, choose the way that is most helpful to you.

You will probably find that the birth plan evolves as the birth approaches. You may alter your plan after reading something online or in a book or talking with someone who plants a seed that flowers into an idea you wish to pursue. For example, you may decide you want only a few private hours with your baby after birth, but while holding your baby, you change your mind and want him with you the entire time. You may want your family and close friends to meet him, too. Or you may think you'll use the hospital-provided gown to dress your baby, then one day you read that many organizations make dresses and outfits from used wedding dresses and you want one for your child. Keep an open mind and make changes as you see fit. These will be important hours that you'll cherish forever. If you intend to make the most of your precious time, you'll probably be grateful that you kept an open mind.

If you wish for the medical team to understand and follow your plan, you may want it clearly written and more formal. In this case, you will probably want someone to make sure your caregiving team sees it prior to your admittance, if possible. It can be mailed or faxed to the head or charge nurse in labor and delivery, to the social work department, and even to your doctor. Too many parents and birth planning advisors have reported that the plan got lost, so providing multiple people with copies and keeping some in your hospital bag may prevent this from happening.

If you are the kind of person who prefers to be informed and needs some control (not a bad thing at all), you may even wish to keep backup ideas in mind (and in your plan) so that the staff have some ideas about how to be supportive. For example, if you intend to have your partner with you, but he travels quite a bit and could be out of town when the time comes, have a backup person listed. If you expect a vaginal birth and a baby who is alive for a while, be aware that a caesarean is possible or that the baby could die before birth. You may wish to discuss what you would do in those situations.

However, if that sounds too difficult and you are able to go with the flow, then your birth plan may be more broad-brush ideas. For example, "I want as many family members as possible there," or "Ask my partner and sister to decide if I can't, since I trust that they know what I would prefer." One tip we have learned is to create a sign or a word that you use with your partner, doula, Baby Loss Family Advisor, or nurse that conveys a message like "Stop. Slow down. I can't take any more." It could also mean "I need some privacy. Get everyone out of the room." Perhaps it is a sign that you make with your hands or a word that you wouldn't normally use, such as your childhood nickname, a foreign word you like, or even a word like "ocean" or "pinecone." Put it in writing on your plan and share it with a birth advocate or family member.

With the birth of a healthy child, some preferences cannot be accommodated due to policies, protocol, or the staff's judgment. However, often in cases where mothers are delivering a baby with a poor or fatal condition, doctors and midwives understand that the birth is a very crucial event for the parents and they often agree to delay routines that are not urgent. This is why it is important to talk to your doctor and midwife about your wishes for birth prior to the hospital admittance, whenever possible. Hopefully, you can agree on what can be done or delayed to make this time special for you.

There are often many parts in a comprehensive birth plan, and they do not need to be discussed or developed in any particular order.

WHY CREATE A BIRTH PLAN?

As a mom of a baby who has special needs or a fatal condition, a birth plan is your way to help ensure that what you would like included is possible. Since you probably have some time prior to birth, it gives you a chance to share your birth plan with your caregivers and your family. With proper preparation and discussion, you will increase your chances of realizing many of your hopes and plans for the birth and its aftermath, such as spending time with your baby.

A birth plan is a tool to help you regain some control after having lost so much with the news that your baby will not be healthy and may in fact die. Although you can't change that, you can at least influence how you give birth and how you care for and spend time with your baby.

The birth plan is also a communication tool, a document with lists and suggestions to give to your doctor or midwife. Since it outlines what you would or would not like to happen during your labor and your preferences under various other circumstances, it offers them much-needed guidance. They want to support you in the best way possible. You help not only yourselves, but your caregivers who want to support you with such a plan.

WHAT IF THE BIRTH PLAN ISN'T FOLLOWED?

Having the birth plan helps you gain some—but not all—control. However, rarely does the formal birth plan go as expected. That is why we refer to a birth plan as *flexible* or as a "birth vision." Most things in life aren't perfect, and birth is definitely one of them. To that end, you'll need to release some of the control and not pin all your hopes on your birth plan. You have let others know what you hope for and allow them to do their best to acknowledge your wishes and ensure that they are accommodated whenever possible. But what if the baby does not come as planned and you need a caesarean? What if your parents are out of town and don't make it for the birth? What if you need more medication than you planned for and you have a memory lapse? What if someone forgot the video camera? What if your doctors are not there or they lose the birth plan? Have contingency plans and problem solve as much as you can during the event. However, still things may change. In the end, the birth will go as it goes. Give yourself permission to allow that to happen. You may wish to pray about it and ask for courage and trust. You may also need to say to yourself and to your partner that you will do all you can and then seek grace and peace.

MEETING AND PARENTING YOUR BABY

In this section of your birth plan you should discuss the care and options available to you and your baby after the birth. You may want to discuss measures to be taken (or not taken) to revive your baby, pain relief available to your child, where your baby will be (the neonatal intensive care unit, in another hospital that can offer a higher degree of care, in your room, or at home with you as soon as possible).

What palliative measures do you seek? Some might include:

- *Medication* (or no medication) for tolerable pain. For high levels of pain, medication that does not cause amnesia.
- *Parenting time* spent bathing and caring for your baby whether alive or not.
- *Breastfeeding or bottle feeding* babies who are alive and able to suck.

- *Holding the baby* the entire time he is alive. Some parents plan for family members to take turns holding baby the while he is alive. Other parents want to be the only ones to hold him while he is alive, allowing other family members to hold him after he dies. You ultimately get to decide, but it would be nice to ask your close family and friends what they are hoping for so that you can take that into consideration.

- *Medical care* for your baby, including the point at which you might stop medical care and ask for tubes and needles to be removed so that you can have quality time alone with your child if she is destined to die.

- *Ideas for saying good-bye.* If you are ready, it might be appropriate to think about ways of saying good-bye now. If you are not, there is no immediate need to do so now. However, it is a good idea to ask others for help with practical preparations. For example, you could ask others to research cemeteries, funeral gowns, and funeral homes with experience working compassionately with small babies. If you aren't ready to hear that information, at least you will know the information is there for you when you are ready.

- *Pictures of your child and your family.* It's a good idea to have cameras available and pictures taken. You may not get another opportunity to take pictures of your child while alive, should he die before you leave the hospital. However, we encourage you, if you feel comfortable, to take pictures of your baby even after he has passed away. Many families also take pictures at the service. You have only a few days to take a lifetime's worth of pictures; make the most of it, even if you are uncomfortable.

- *Dressing your baby* may be a comfort to you, so take a special outfit or clothing to the hospital with you. Dressing and caring for your baby in this way can be comforting. Many hospitals have gowns and blankets, so check if you want to learn about their resources.

- *Make arrangements for religious or other special rituals* that can be performed in the hospital. Many hospitals have religious staff on-site who can perform a blessing or baptism, along with offering prayers.

- *Sharing healing stories* will provide a lifelong comfort to you and your family. Many people don't think about other family members, who will also grieve and who may have a need to meet and be with your baby.

You will probably think of other ways that you can be the parent to your baby during this important time.

For many parents who have never seen—or expected to see—a dead child and who are probably not even comfortable with dead pets, the idea of meeting your baby and spending time with him may be scary. Don't reject this idea now. Trust that when the time comes and you meet your baby, you will know what to do. Take the advice of countless nurses who have helped families after birth as well as the parents who realized how natural and necessary it was to hold their babies and spend as much precious time with them as they could. Realize like they did that you will get no other opportunities in this lifetime and no "do-overs."

Sue S., a nurse and prenatal specialist, recounts stories about other families' experiences to all her new clients as she birth plans with them. To one couple, she offered as an example the parents who wanted to spend two full days with their baby and described what a wonderful and blessed experience that time was for them. That sounded odd to the father with whom she was birth planning, and he stated that he could not imagine spending so much time with the baby. He felt that a few minutes would be sufficient. However, this father ultimately spent three days with his baby. He could not have predicted what he wanted or needed during birth planning, but given support and the option to wait and see, he felt grateful to have had his child with him in the hospital room for three full days.

CREATING AND COLLECTING MEMENTOS AND RITUALS

Sometimes staff want to help *and* they want to protect you. They may take your baby out of the room to bathe him or to cut a lock of hair or to dress her. Although this might seem helpful, they are parenting your baby and taking away your opportunities to do it. You may want to specify that you want to do the parenting but will ask for help if needed. Ideally, they should honor your wishes. There are many ways you can be involved with your baby and collect mementos, memories, and ritu- als. These are further explored in chapter 10, "Memory Creation."

Remember to include your close family and friends during this time. Shared memories of your baby will be important in the days ahead. If you do it without them, they won't have special memories and won't be able to remember your precious baby with you—how she felt, how much she weighed, who she looked like, what was said as she was loved up by her family, and so much more.

> We did not know any better, but we sure made some mistakes and hold many regrets even three decades later. We wonder why we didn't invite Brennan's grandparents to the hospital to meet him before we had him cremated. Our siblings were starving to help and be a part of it, too, and we didn't include them in anything where he was present. They never saw him, and even if we had pictures— which we don't—it is not the same as being there and holding him.
> —Sherokee

There are many books and other resources to help give you ideas. The web is full of them; we've included a few for your review in the back of this book.

BABY LOSS DOULAS/FAMILY ADVISORS

A new paradigm of care for families has emerged to assist women and their partners through the birth of a baby, including slowing things down and getting help creating the birth plan. Baby Loss Family Advis- ors, sometimes also called Baby Loss Doulas, bereavement doulas, or care companions, are well trained to help during this time, especially with creating or evaluating birth plans.

Loss Advisors/Loss Doulas also may be available as companions dur- ing the birth; they can assist with keepsake creation; they can help parents understand their rights; they even can inform and help parents bring their babies home after death; and they can offer support over time. They are also aware of relevant resources to assist bereaved par- ents. A list of qualified Loss Advisors is available from the website www.babylossfamilyadvisor.org.

APPROACHING THE DATE OF BIRTH

As you get closer to your baby's due date, you may have mixed feelings. You may feel regretful that it will soon be over. As one mom put it, "Each day we are closer to the due date is one less day with my baby boy." This is your time together. Even though there may be medical issues or health threats, there is a sense of safety with having your baby in your womb. Soon everything will change.

Prior to the birth, you may want to collect as many pre-birth mementos as you can. From the doctor appointment notes, to copies of your chart, to any notes or announcements you sent out, to sonogram pictures or videos—these items can be kept in a special place; perhaps later they will go in a chest or a memory box.

> Last week we had the baby's 3D/4D ultrasound picture taken by a volunteer who gives these sessions away for free to moms like me. She gave us printed pictures, a CD full of still pictures, and even a recorded DVD with the entire session on video. The pictures are amazing and I look at him every day. Having the photo session done made for such a positive bonding experience. I loved watching him move and am beyond grateful we have it recorded on DVD, especially since the doctors assume he will be stillborn. Being able to watch him move on the video when he might not get the chance [to] after delivery is a great gift. It was incredible charity! —Toni-Marie

Do not let third parties including family, friends, and hospital staff convince you about what is best for you or your child unless it genuinely feels right. Birthing in a hospital can be very cold and clinical. Although you may feel overwhelmed by the setting and be under the impression that you are a "guest" in someone else's house, remember that you are the parents of your precious little one and that the staff are there to support you.

Don't let fear of the unknown ruin this important window of time. Remember, you loved this baby while alive; you still love this baby who happens to have died or has serious issues. Let that love drive your time together.

Here is a sample birth plan created by Toni-Marie and her husband after reading a draft of this chapter. The staff did their best to follow it, finding it extremely helpful, and Toni-Marie and her husband went to the hospital with a calmness knowing they had a birth vision.

EXAMPLE OF A BIRTH PLAN

Birth Plan
BIRTH DAY, our way

Baby: John Carl

Mom's Name: <u>T.M. V.</u>

Doctor's Name: <u>Dr. W. F.</u>

Due Date: _____

Hospital/Birth Center: <u>Regional Medical Center</u>

* Only allow *immediate* family and their spouses in for visitation. All outside guests such as friends and nonfamily members are asked to respect our privacy.

DURING LABOR:

Permit my husband (A. V.) and my mother (P. A.) to be present at all times.

If my caregiver is not available, we would like a doctor/midwife who is familiar with and supportive of natural childbirth methods, as well as being aware of our particular situation.

Let labor begin on its own.

I wish to be alert and involved in my baby's labor and birth. Pain medication may be asked for, *but not any that causes amnesia*.

My preferences about medication are: At this time we are open to using an epidural because we feel the heartache of the baby's passing will be painful enough.

Do not offer me drugs to accelerate labor. I will request them if I want them.

Provide only intermittent fetal monitoring.

I've had three episiotomies in the past so I am open to one again.

We would like the freedom to choose a delivery position.

We would like to bring our own music and scents.

AFTER BIRTH:

My husband <u>A. V.</u> will cut the umbilical cord.

After birth, immediately place the baby onto my abdomen.

If John Carl is born alive, permit breastfeeding only—no bottles, pacifiers, or formula.

We would like our baby to be given directly to Mom for nursing and cuddling.

If death is expected, we would like our baby to not receive any unnecessary procedures, such as blood tests, [others listed here], except for pain relief, if needed.

However, if initial care of the baby is mandatory, we request it be done while baby is on my body.

Allow in-rooming with baby, and perform all exams of baby in our presence.

We want our other children to see the baby while alive, and we would like some family photos.

We would appreciate some time alone if our baby has passed away, as well as if our baby is not going to survive so that we can say our hellos and good-byes.

We would like our baby to be treated with the utmost respect, including after death.

We have contacted [I just cannot bring myself to contact anyone yet] funeral director who will be transporting our baby to the funeral home.

MEMORY CREATION:

We wish to have a photographer come to our room. We would appreciate your support in giving us privacy for this.

We wish to bathe our baby, though we may ask for help.

We have been given a memory box full of items for memory making, and we would like to take our baby's blanket home with us.

We would like to cut some of our baby's hair for a memento.

We would like hand- and footprints done, three-dimensional would be lovely if possible.

We are still thinking about videotaping time with baby; let's keep the option open.

7

THE LABOR AND BIRTH

The birth of a child is an intense experience for any parent. Bringing life into the world, no matter how fragile it may seem, is a humbling experience both physically and emotionally. As you have chosen to carry your precious child to term, you may be overwhelmed with questions, doubts, and fears about the labor and birth of your baby. That is understandable. You have so much to consider. If you have not given birth before, you will want to refer to childbirth preparation for more specifics about the stages of labor.

THE POSSIBILITIES

It is possible that your baby may die prior to birth. Most parents express their deep desire to meet their babies alive and to have some special time together before she dies. This does not always happen, however. You have probably been forewarned that some babies die prior to birth. This is called a stillbirth. Although we don't want you to stress about it—and we hope you realize your dream of time with your baby while still alive—we feel that it is important to help you know your rights and options if your baby dies during pregnancy or delivery.

If this were to happen, remember that you still have many of the same rights and expectations during labor and after birth as you would if your baby is alive. You have rights, for example, to have pain relief, to choose your labor position, to ask questions, and to have family members present to support you during labor and birth. The staff who will be assisting you will be supporting you and hopefully will be respectful of you, just as they would for any other family. You have the right to experience this birth as peacefully as possible. The key, however, is to know this and to make sure you can be assertive regarding your needs at all stages of pregnancy, labor, and birth. Communicate those needs to the staff or appoint someone to speak on your behalf.

You can seek a natural birth, though you may be encouraged to take more medication than you wish. Stay strong and tell them what you truly want, even if you do need some pain medication. You can still spend time with your baby and have family near you. So much of the following will still apply. The time you spend with baby is very precious and memorable. Even though it is disappointing to have your baby die sooner than you hoped, make the most of this time. As we say often, you get no do-overs here. Even with a stillborn child, you may swaddle and hold your baby, and you may take pictures and spend time with him. You may bathe and sit with your baby. Whatever you decide you want to do is up to you in most cases, and your wishes should be clearly conveyed to personnel. If you feel that you need someone to speak on your behalf, ask someone whom you trust or even write down your wishes. And if you change your mind, that is fine, too. You may want to address your thoughts and concerns to medical staff and family members even while your baby is still alive in utero, in case something changes and you need to make decisions on the fly.

And if your baby is born alive—whether he lives for an hour, a day, or longer—you will want his birth to be special and full of warm memories. The physical birth itself may be fairly normal or it may have complications. Your care provider should be able to explain what is likely to happen. For example, if there is worry about whether the baby can be born naturally due to some of the problems or the positioning of the child, you would want to know about caesarean delivery and how and when you might know if that becomes a serious option. A C-section may be necessary in any event; this happens with many deliveries, as well as if complications arise during labor and delivery.

The emotional side of this birth will be particularly intense. Unfortunately, the birth of your child may represent his or her death, the beginning of lifelong care, or further uncertainty.

The fact that the midwives were so nice toward Lana and kept saying how gorgeous she was (although she had both spina bifida and Down syndrome) allowed us to express love and emotions toward our baby. In a sense, we felt it was okay she wasn't "perfect." —Lana's mom

PAIN RELIEF

You may want to explore natural birth or whether you want any pain medication. There are some stronger medications that may result in fogginess. Many moms express sadness or even anger that they were given medication that knocked them out or caused them to have little or no memory of the birth and the time they spent with their babies after birth. The hospital staff may offer you these drugs to protect you, so that you don't feel pain or get too emotional. Yet they may not have prepared you for the downside. In some deliveries, after a baby is born, the mom may need further surgery if complications arise, and anesthesia may be administered in an emergency situation. You may tell your medical staff ahead of time that if that happens, you would like your baby to remain in your room or available to you when you awake. You will want to remember those first precious minutes of birth and of holding your child; therefore, you may wish to opt for the more common medications, such as an epidural (which may numb your lower extremities) or other pain medication that provides some pain relief but allows you to remain fairly alert. You will have so little time with your baby in a physical sense if your baby dies or will die shortly. Have this important conversation with your physician and also with your partner, make your decision, then be sure to communicate it prior to labor, directly to your care provider. Preparation and awareness about your options and preferences can provide peace. If during delivery you opt for medications, that is fine, too. Just be sure to relay your wishes to your team.

There are three main forms of pain relief in labor: systemic medication, local anesthesia, and natural/nonmedical pain relief. Depending upon your situation and even the country you live in, you may be able to choose any of them or even combine them. Understand that you have the right to feel comfortable both physically and emotionally while also meeting your other objective of meeting your baby in an alert state.

I told my nurse I did not want to feel pain. What I did not say out loud is that I did want to see and remember my baby's birth and our skin-to-skin time together right after birth. And no one asked me that question. As it turned out, when I really came out of the deep haze was many hours later. The birth had taken place, the baby had been brought to the NICU for evaluation, and then had died without me present. Why did I have to get medication that put me in such a fog? No matter how hard I try I can't remember anything about that time. I can't forgive myself or my doctor. Those precious minutes are gone and I don't get a second chance with my daughter. —Anonymous

Systemic Medication

Systemic medication (e.g., morphine) is administered via the mother's bloodstream (intravenously) or more commonly through muscle (intramuscularly). The known adverse effects are vomiting, nausea, itching, and sleepiness for both the mother and the baby. One of the potential outcomes of morphine, especially if a medium to heavy dose is used, is that it may cause fogginess. Many mothers who have used morphine report that they don't remember much about the labor or birth; others report being present though perhaps a bit foggy while receiving morphine or other similar medications. There may be a fog and some vague or blank times that can't be accounted for, making it difficult for some to recapture what happened. This may or may not happen and is experienced differently by individual women.

I was given morphine during labor. It did not cause amnesia in my situation. I remembered almost everything. —A mom

Another medication is the well-known laughing gas (Entonox), which is a mixture of nitrous oxide and oxygen. Mothers apply a mask to their faces and breathe the mixture at each contraction. Your midwife or doctor will be able to discuss this form of pain relief with you.

Local Anesthesia

The local anesthesia used most commonly during childbirth is known as an epidural, which involves injecting a combination of drugs including a narcotic and an anesthetic into the lower back to reduce pain. An epidural prevents the spinal nerves from receiving pain messages. Some of the adverse effects on the mother are numbness, shivering, ringing in the ears, nausea, a temporary inability to control bodily functions, an inability to move the lower body or walk, and backaches, as well as potential for headaches that occasionally can be severe. If you have taken birthing classes, you may have actually seen the equipment used to give women epidurals. It is one of the most commonly utilized pain medications offered and used during delivery. Many women opt for an epidural even for deliveries of healthy babies. Most doctors recommend that pregnant women take this route. Most women report no feelings of mental fog or amnesia with epidurals. This might be a good option, as it minimizes pain while allowing presence of mind and the ability to immediately hold and connect with a newborn.

Natural Methods

Many natural methods have been developed over the years to control pain during labor. Some have not been proven, while others are renowned for their efficacy.

You may or may not want to try natural pain relief, but you have the right to attempt those that you think will be helpful. Your doctor or midwife will be able to help you with questions that you may have about the following methods of natural pain relief.

- Aromatherapy is a process of relaxation that involves the use of oils and scents in the labor room.
- Hypnotherapy puts the mother-to-be into a deep trance so that she cannot feel pain.
- The Lamaze technique is a practical method for helping the mother to relax through breathing exercises and understanding her body and the labor process.
- Bathing in warm water is often used to help the mother-to-be to relax.
- Acupuncture involves the use of needles to diminish pain and to help the mother relax.
- TENS (transcutaneous electronic nerve stimulation) is a procedure that involves the application of electrical receptors to specif-

ic parts of the body to moderate pain. It is usually administered by
a trained professional.

- Touch or massage is a widespread approach that has been used
  for centuries. It involves having a birth partner massage the mother's back, neck, feet, or legs during labor.
- Maternal movement and position change have been recognized as
  facilitating the labor process. Mothers are encouraged to walk and
  move around.

Labor and birth are an important part of the process toward parenthood. You will tell this story repeatedly. Be thoughtful about your
choices, knowing that your baby may not live outside the womb or for
very long. Each moment that you have and each choice that you make
can be viewed as sacred and special. Look deep within yourself to
decide what is important to you at this special time.

TIPS AND ADVICE

- Inquire about antenatal classes, particularly if this is your first baby.
  What kind of classes does your hospital offer? Can you access them
  one on one if you prefer not to see other pregnant women?
- What kind of birth model does your birth facility offer? Midwife led?
  Ob-gyn led? Can you bring in a support person such as a doula or
  family advocate/advisor?
- Start thinking about pain relief options. Do you have a preference?
  Do you understand them all? If not, who can you ask about it?
- Have you decided and planned your birth ambiance? Would you like
  soft music, candles, or a particular sheet or blanket on you? Make
  sure to discuss options with your birth attendant and bring those
  items along with you. A word of caution, though, whatever ambiance
  you create will stay with you forever. Be careful about choosing pop-
  ular songs that you could hear after the birth, as they will trigger
  memories.
- Do you have a camera (and a photographer, whether a professional
  or family member) and a way to videotape the birth and its aftermath? Pictures are wonderful, but parents tell us there is nothing like

a video of people holding your baby, hearing the loving words that are spoken, and, if you are fortunate, seeing your baby move.

- Who will be your birth partner? Have you discussed what would be helpful (e.g., massages, ice, silence, words, touching, etc.) with this person? Does this person feel confident or does he or she have questions? Who could he or she ask? Are you able to have other family members at the delivery? If so, who do you want there? When do you want them to leave?
- Be open-minded about how things develop. Birth is a unique experience and sometimes things go as planned. At other times, they do not and that's okay. Be prepared for a special journey knowing that some things will be decided at the last minute.

8

IF YOUR BABY IS BORN ALIVE

Like almost all parents in your situation, you want your child to live for at least a while after birth. As you consider your options and the future outcome of this pregnancy, you may have been given different ideas about whether your baby would live after birth. Maybe she will live a short while or she could have a longer life. Not knowing makes it hard to plan and to have a sense of what your hopes should and could be.

BEING WITH YOUR BABY

Explore your options for being with your baby based on the present situation, not only on the birth plan you made. Talk with the staff about how things will go regarding the amount of time you want to spend with your baby. You can make plans to hold, bathe, dress, and parent your child. Don't be afraid of hurting your baby, a common fear. It is highly unlikely you can hurt her, but do talk about it with your caregivers. This is your chance for cuddling and skin-to-skin contact. Changing your baby's diapers and combing her hair are some of the active parenting tasks you can do. Ask staff what mementos they will help you create and talk with your family about their involvement. Remember to include your family so that they can meet and create their own memories of the baby. Over time, this shared memory will give you all special times to talk about it.

Although it may seem foreign to you, most—though not all—hospital staff understand the need for parents to meet and be with their babies before saying good-bye. The baby loss community has taught them this and there is now research to support it. Options for being with your baby while at the hospital should be discussed prior to the birth.

MEDICAL INTERVENTION

As the doctors assess your baby, they may tell you that she may not live long, so you will be asked about the amount of medical intervention you want. These questions will depend upon the diagnosis and predicted problems your baby has. Have a few conversations with your medical providers about what types of intervention might be available. Dissect the pros and cons of the intervention itself—the value of it and what it means about how you and your family can be with your baby.

As you contemplate this decision, you may wonder if you want the baby to be in the neonatal intensive care unit (NICU) receiving care or next to you (which may limit what can be done medically). Do you want breathing tubes (intubation), extra testing, surgery, and other life-sustaining procedures? Or do you want your baby to remain in your (and your families') arms so you can hold your baby for the rest of her life?

Tracy Ahrens shares in her book *Giant Hero* that she did not see her son Titus much after he was born. "I couldn't be with him because I was so tired. I had just given birth. I couldn't feel my legs. I was numb from the epidural. I was also afraid to see Titus like that, with tubes and things coming out of him." Then he was transferred to a Chicago hospital NICU and she writes, "When I saw Titus in Chicago I was so angry. There were way more tubes and things in him than I ever wanted. I did not want to have to deal with turning off any life support machines." Despite your best efforts, things can get out of hand. You may discover decisions are made and care is given that you are uncomfortable with, which can lead to anger and frustration. Hopefully, this won't happen to you, but if it does, seek help from others—the hospital's social worker, other family members, your faith advisor, or friends who work in the medical field who can help you navigate. This is also a perfect opportunity to find a perinatal hospice/Baby Loss Family Advisor who can guide you and intervene where necessary on your behalf.

Some parents choose no intervention, recognizing that they can then hold their baby for his entire life, given that he will die anyway. However, there may be reasons why some intervention may be your choice. For instance, maybe you want to wait for family to arrive and you hope to keep the baby alive until they arrive. Maybe you feel the baby is suffering and you want some pain medication administered. Or maybe you believe that your baby can survive and you want medical staff to do everything possible to help him. In any case, after consultation with your doctor, your partner, and perhaps your faith supporters, you will come to a decision that works for you. And if you change your mind, you still may be able to do things differently. This will be a time of personal reflection as you work toward a decision that you both feel good about. Barring specific hospital rules, you should be the one to decide how these final hours, days, or longer go with your baby.

> I feel so good that I can say my baby was held his entire life . . . in my womb and then he was lovingly passed from one family member to another the entire time he lived. I have no regrets about that. —Anonymous

> We are fighters and our baby was a fighter. We felt it was our job to do everything we could for her while she was alive. Watching her in the NICU with all the tubes, tests, and equipment was very hard. We just wanted to hold her. But as a result we got ten extra days with her and we'll forever be grateful. After she died, we held her for hours. It was hard, but so good to finally examine her, love her up, and have some skin-to-skin time. —A mom

WHAT ARE THE SIGNS THAT THE BABY MAY BE DYING?

As your time with baby draws to a close, a few things happen that you may wish to know. You may worry about the dying process, so being prepared for what might happen can help inform and calm you. As a parent, it will be hard to watch if you think your baby is in pain, so you might want to talk about pain relief. Your child's body may begin to cool as his systems shut down and the oxygen lessens. Lethargy and listlessness might occur. Talk with your caregivers, who should have experience with babies who die, especially if they work in the NICU. They will probably tell you that, depending upon your baby's issues, there may be some breathing difficulties or breathing slows. Your baby may begin to change color, often turning bluish for lack of oxygen. And his lips might become more reddish. Don't be surprised if there are some sighing or crying sounds; a few gasps may even occur. On the other hand, some babies breathe shallowly for a while and then their heart stops, which may not be obvious to those watching. Some parents share their feelings of love with their baby and then give them permission to go. Interestingly, a number of parents recount that shortly after being given this message, their babies take a last breath. Read more about this in chapter 9, "If Your Baby Dies."

> Our young son wanted to constantly check his sister's heart rate as she slowly died. He would kiss and touch her, talk about how cute she was, and then would check her heart rate. "I still hear it," he would say. After a few hours, he looked up at us and said, "Mommy, I think she left." It was something that he could do; months and years later he still felt proud of how he helped us and her at that time. —A mom

BABY LIVES

There are cases, no matter what the tests or doctors predict, when the baby may not die as quickly as was originally thought. And in fact, sometimes the baby lives for a short or even long time. It is important to know that there are no guarantees about this. Some babies fight very hard to live. One mother was told by her doctor that her baby would die shortly after being taken off life support, yet he lived for eleven more hours. During that time mom, dad, and family members passed the baby to each other and held him the entire time. Music played, stories were told, and amazing memories were created.

There is a Facebook page for a group calling itself "End 'Incompatible with Life,'" and it suggests that using that phrase deceives parents into thinking that their baby will *surely* die, usually within the first minutes or hours of life. Yet many parents have found that they were not prepared for how to deal with their baby who lived—some with severe problems and some with issues far less dire than predicted. If this is the case for you, you'll need to know what resources are available and get some help with how to proceed. You will find some of these resources at the back of this book.

OPTIONS FOR BRINGING BABY HOME

If it looks like your baby will live, the conversation may turn to bringing him home. Parents who have done this often need advice and help with taking care of their baby with medical needs that might include suctioning his nose, feeding issues, and care for any specific issues the baby may have. Ask questions and watch the staff to learn how to care for your baby. Find out where and how to get any equipment needed and certainly what to watch for as signs of distress or extreme problems.

Some problems may occur that you don't feel prepared to deal with, and there may be times when you feel hospitalization is necessary. You may wonder whom you will call, how you will get the baby there, and what might happen once the baby is back in the hospital. It is wise to get a plan and a written list from your medical provider and hospital staff prior to leaving, including who to call and their number. Also be sure you have instructions in writing, including what to watch for that might be a sign to call for help.

Your original dream of a joyful homecoming with your baby may be significantly altered when you actually bring your sick or disabled baby home. On the other hand, as you adjust your dreams and expectations, you may find that the amount of time with your baby may be more than you expected. You may find you even have feelings of gratefulness at this time. The emotions, which can include grief and loss, will need to be dealt with at some time, though perhaps not now. It's okay to put those feelings on hold as you cope and survive. As you bring your baby home, you'll want to focus on your child's well-being. You may experience doubts, questions, and anxiety about how to care for your child, as well as concerns about the future and your ability to cope. Many parents have said that their first reaction was to ask themselves whether they would be able to do it. Would they know how to take care of the baby's special needs? Would they do things "right"? What if their baby dies at home? How will they prepare for this and cope during such stressful times?

There is no magical pill or answer that will take away those normal concerns, but knowing that they are common and reading about how others managed the transition may help. Parents who are about to take a special needs baby home need to know as much as possible about their child's condition. It is important to focus on what your baby will need immediately upon coming home as opposed to what he will need as time goes on. That time will come. You may need to focus on the present issues now.

Maybe your baby needs special equipment such as special sleeping monitors, strollers, high chairs, or feeding tools. The hospital's neonatologist or social worker will inform you about what you need to organize and prepare. Another source of information and support can be found through your public or private pediatrician, community nurse, local office for independent living, disability support service, or other relevant specialist. It is very unlikely that the hospital will discharge you without putting you in contact with the appropriate medical specialists. You will be able to learn about your child's needs gradually as you go forward.

> There were no considerations or adjustments needed straight away for Jared. The only thing we did was put air conditioning [on in] the car. It was a stifling summer and we would get him out of his car seat and his head would be saturated. —Kylie

You may anticipate that your baby may pass away at home. If this is the case, we would advise you to have a plan that will help you prepare and bring you some calm. Your doctor, your palliative nurse, or your social worker will be able to work with you on this plan. However, do talk to your doctor about your baby's specific condition and needs, keep a list of contact numbers in case of emergency, and prepare emotionally for when that time comes. You will need to know how long you can keep your baby with you at home; if you need to call a funeral director, emergency personnel, police, a doctor, or someone else; what rights you have; how much time you have with your baby before having to let him go to the funeral home; and who will help you plan a funeral or other end-of-life event if you choose to have one. Hopefully, having some of those decisions in place will help you embrace your baby's passing, surrounded by peace and loved ones. More is written about this in chapter 11, "Saying Good-bye."

To help you keep on top of what is happening with your baby, we suggest that you keep a notebook in a specific place, like the kitchen or next to the baby's crib, so you can refer to your notes and add information about the care you are giving or any symptoms you see. At times like this your memory will abandon you or play tricks. Stress can do that, so use other tools such as writing it down, putting it in your phone memo, or asking a friend to help you remember. It is also wise to have an observer with you when you talk with the doctor.

COPING

If your child lives for a while—or a long time—you will develop coping strategies, find ways that work best for you, and hopefully experience some really special family moments to cherish. It may be important for you to find others who have had a child with similar issues—your medical provider may be able to provide names. The web lists organizations where you can connect with others and even social media sites like Facebook may offer you group-chat opportunities. Just be careful about how much you rely on others you don't know to give you advice. If that advice is of a medical nature, you may want to check it out with your doctor. Emotional support and sharing resources are two of the most wonderful things about connecting with others facing similar outlooks with their children. At least you will feel less alone and you'll be surrounded and supported by others who "get it."

PHOTOS AND VIDEOS

You will never forget bringing your baby home. But as time goes by, you may forget the color of specific outfits, who was at your home, the cute things your baby did, what the weather was like when you took your baby out for the first time, or who she resembled during those first hours. You could create a personal photo album for your baby with some of the highlights of her life. Those may include friends, family, or inspiring moments. Take videos; there is nothing like seeing people move and speak. Don't be shy; there are never too many memories!

Your baby will grow and change. This time is very precious. Some parents suggest that you take a photo every day so that you have nice reminders of your baby's changes over time. If it looks like your child may live much longer, you may wish to do it weekly or monthly. Parents have suggested that taking the photo in the same position or next to the same object (such as a teddy bear or in their crib) helps to highlight changes, show size, and provide continuity. Of course, taking pictures of your baby with other family members is extremely important. Including your other living children—or even nieces and nephews—can be helpful to them at the time and over time, when their memories fade. Younger children may actually have no memories at all, so pictures and videos can help tell the story. These pictures will help them hold some memory and know that they were involved with their sibling while she was still alive. You will cherish all those photos in the days ahead.

LIVING MEMORY BOX

Create a memory box and put special things in it from the earliest days. As time goes on, you can continue adding to it. You could store anything from the first outfit, to the name of the first visitor you receive, special books that you read, tickets to the zoo, fall leaves, your children's drawings, cards you receive, letters you write to your baby, and so much more. The contents will become tangible memories of special moments from your baby's life. You will be reminded of all that she brought into your life and to be able to show others, including subsequent children, when the time is right.

> I kept Lana's first picture on the fridge for years. . . . For so long, I never thought she'd write or draw like that. . . . Now it's in her baby box, but it's still very precious. —Lana's mom

> Although Talina passed away twelve years ago now, I kept all the research papers and articles I have written on the topic of prenatal diagnosis in her baby box. Because for me, those are not my achievements. They are hers. —Stephanie

THE GIFTS

You cannot predict how long your baby will be with you. However, no matter how long it is, it will never be long enough. Hopefully, you will have many experiences with your child and you will see the positive gifts that will change you and others. You may look at life differently and realize how important relationships are, given life's fragility. These are gifts that come from, and because of, your baby. Maybe his little life touched someone deeply and they are changed in profound ways. Many families become altruistic, creating a legacy that lives on. Parents may start or participate in a run or walk that honors their baby. Some join organizations, start websites, and donate baby items or self-help materials to other families in need. Your baby's short life can become a springboard for any number of gifts as you seek your new normal and learn to see beauty and love in the world in a new way. Your attitude and behavior may change in amazing ways.

> I do live my life differently now, better really. Sunsets, flowers, beauty, love, joy, time with my children and family . . . they all seem to matter more now. I do not take life for granted and I do my best to live life fully. It is a miracle when things go well. I credit the short lives of my babies for waking me up to this new attitude. —Sherokee

SELF-CARE

Self-care is important for moms after giving birth and for supportive dads. It is especially important while caring for a child with special needs or while you await your baby's death if that is imminent. There are a number of helpful suggestions for taking care of yourself in chapter 22, "Postpartum and Self-care," but a few specific ones are provided here.

TIME TO YOURSELF

Bringing any baby home results in busyness! It can be even more busy and stressful when your baby has special needs or is unwell. However, if you're able to give yourself at least a half hour a day to yourself, it will help. The time could be used to reflect, to think about your dreams and life, to read or exercise, or to do nothing at all. Remember that you just gave birth, and your body is healing. Call in family members or friends to help—accept their offers to cook dinner or take your other children out for an afternoon so that you can get much-needed rest. Try to establish a routine for yourself that includes taking care of yourself: eating regular meals, getting some sunlight every day, sleeping and resting as much as you need, and finding help with the housework (or just forget it for now!). Schedule follow-up care with your doctor, and seek out mental health professionals if you feel that you need emotional support that you're not currently getting.

TIME OUT

For some babies born with a life-altering prenatal diagnosis, their conditions will not be life threatening. For other babies, their prognosis may provide them with a limited lifespan. Either way, it is not humanly possible to live on standby for months or years; you may need to remind yourself that your relationship, your family, your social life, and even your studies or career should continue to be important to you. Ask family members or a paid babysitter to help watch the children so you can get an occasional break, if possible. Do what you can to find some normalcy in your day and your life. Though this isn't always possible, with a will to try and with help from others, you may find a way.

TIME WITH YOUR PARTNER

Go out on dates with your partner, if you have one. Plan ahead and do your best to stick to your scheduled dates. You can divide your date into the "fun part" (no child or serious subjects talk), where you play, laugh, dance, or go to a movie. Then if you wish to use some of this one-on-one time—and because you know you can't help yourself—choose a time frame, such as twenty minutes, to talk family business. A date without family business and baby subjects would be a good goal to seek.

GOING FORWARD

Your life has changed. It may be difficult in some ways and really special in other ways. In any case, each person in your family will have to adapt to the changes that come with a baby who has special needs. Explore the resources and the people who can help you now. You will need to build your network as you go forward.

You can't see what is ahead and you won't know how your child will do over time. Maybe she will improve and her life will become a steady state where there is some routine and calm. Or maybe your child will need continuous medical or emotional care.

If you have other children, stay in touch with how they are doing. Listen to what they say and look at what they draw. Talk with their teachers about how things are going in school. Change and stress impacts everyone in your home and in your extended family, to some degree. When tough times come, as they will, see them as temporary and go back to your community for support and help. Do not try to do this alone. Find the support you need from your doctors, counselors, faith advisors/clergy, and family. You will need courage and strength along with patience. Believe that you can do this and play that part to the degree you can. Positive attitudes and actions can go a long way to help you move ahead.

9

IF YOUR BABY DIES

If your baby dies prior to birth or shortly after birth, your emotions will run high. Even if you knew this could happen, perhaps you hoped and prayed it wouldn't. Shock still takes over and emotions run high. If you have had time to do some planning, you may have more control. Maybe you made family plans to bring a live baby home, even for a few hours. Maybe you thought your child would live long enough to meet your relatives and be held by you all. This means your dreams and expectations have been dashed. You may feel cheated and deeply disappointed. Sadness and shock may still overwhelm you. Yet your first priority will be to *be with your baby*. This is a time to determine who you want near you and how much alone time you need with your baby. Also, don't rush out the door of the hospital unless you arrange to take your baby with you. This is your time together with those who can guide and support you. You get so little time together with your child and you get no do-overs.

Maybe you have already created a birth plan and talked with the hospital prior to the labor and birth about what you want to happen (see more on this in chapter 6, "Birth Plans and Preparation"). If you have not done this or have an informal plan, you'll still want to communicate your wishes for birth and being with your baby. And if your baby has already died, you can take a few hours or a day to gain some control and make those plans. There are some babies who die during labor; these are the times when planning may not have yet happened, so you go with the flow. Preparing (if you feel able) makes it easier when you meet your child. More and more parents seek a self-reliant role, rather than leaving the power and decision making to other family members or the staff.

As you will read in the next chapter, you will want to spend time making memories, creating rituals, and being present with your baby after the birth. This is the time you have to make "mountains out of moments" prior to saying good-bye. After all, this is all the time you have to meet and make memories of your baby, which will help you over time. Don't be in a rush to be done. Even if you don't want to hold your baby the entire time, maybe others in your family would like their turn.

It has become standard in most developed countries for parents to have their babies with them in their hospital rooms after death. You could spend hours, or even a day or two, with your baby after his death. Yes, there are many families who spend a day or two with their baby after death. This may be your only time to be with your baby after birth if she is born still or even if she lived a while and then died. This is your time, so don't rush it. As parents, you should be the ones to determine how you will *be* with your baby. After all, you are the patient and the parent, and she is *your* child.

Unless your baby has a communicable disease, being with your baby the entire time in the hospital room should be possible. If you get resistance from hospital staff, ask them to show you the policy or the law that restricts your rights. It is possible that they continue restrictive policies based simply on past procedure, not always on what is best for their patients. Ask them to show proof that what you want is not possible.

Spend the time examining and cuddling your child. You may bring in clothes from home and then dress your baby for hours, taking pictures along the way. Many parents invite their other children and extended families to spend time with baby as they parent him by giving him baths, diapering and dressing him, and making handprints and footprints. This could be in the hospital, at the funeral home, or possibly in your own home. Nathalie wrote that she put her daughter on a bed of rose petals, enjoying the intimacy and beauty, then had pictures taken. Make your time really special. Chapter 15, "Holding onto Memories," can help you.

We know that you might find some these ideas scary or unfathomable because you have never heard of anyone doing such a thing or you may have fears about dead bodies. So did we. But that changed once we spent some time with our babies and realized that it wasn't scary at all; rather, it was beautiful and memorable. Looking back, the memories of that time are irreplaceable. Our children were beautiful to us and sharing them with others helps the entire family. Parents cherish their babies and those memories throughout the rest of their lives. Many parents come to realize that they "did not know what they did not know," having made their decisions based on fear or avoidance. They have regrets that they didn't spend enough time with their babies. It is from them that we all have learned to keep suggesting to parents that they take this time with their babies. If, however, after everything—our encouragement and the staff's repeated offers—you chose not to spend prolonged, or any, time with your baby, then don't. And don't feel guilty about it. It is your baby and your decision.

> The official pronouncement of Josh's death came an hour after his delivery, but I'd known he was dead since he'd come out without a pulse. If they'd been able to resuscitate him, someone would have told me. The hospital staff said we could have him for half an hour. What a joke! He was our baby, not theirs. I wish we had been more clear about that and more demanding. —Anonymous

> This is the story of how I said hello to my stillborn son. Not for half an hour like the hospital staff wanted. Not for the six hours I negotiated when they could give me no good reason for the half hour limit. No: this is the story of how I said hello to my stillborn son in the days that followed, in visits to the funeral parlor, in his visits to our home. —Elizabeth Heineman, *Still Life with Baby*

> The time we spent with our baby at home was the most important thing we did. Our children met Olivia and our parents did, too. The private time we had with her was amazing. It could not have happened in the hospital! We are so grateful to our nurse who helped us do this despite the hospital's resistance. —A dad

WHAT TO EXPECT?

You may have some fears or feelings of avoidance; don't let them keep you from being your baby's mother or father. Fear of what he will look like or that he is too fragile to hold are common, as are fears that you will harm your baby or that you might "lose it" while holding him. These are commonly held fears, though not always expressed out loud. These are also the reasons parents often give for not doing what was in their heart: they blame it on those fears. What you want to focus on is that you loved your baby while alive and you still love your baby despite his death. Focus on the love and realize that parents love their children no matter what they look like. Many parents don't even notice birthmarks or discoloration. Lori remembers showing her stillborn daughter's pictures to family and close friends for a few weeks. One day she showed Jenny's picture to her friend Matt. After a few moments, he asked about a dark circle on Jenny's stomach. Lori looked at the spot with shock and said, "I don't know. I have never seen that before."

This is a common occurrence—mothers and fathers often don't see their baby's imperfections. Rather, they see their beloved baby. Even if you do notice the marks or discoloration, it's fine. There will be some parents who find it difficult or bittersweet to see their child. Some of it may be because they are angry or upset. Or it could be that seeing a baby who has problems is hard and painful. That doesn't mean you love your baby less. Sometimes it helps to notice everything about your child.

Share your plans with family and staff for caring for your baby's body, self-transport, funeral plans, and even for time at home with your baby, if regional, local, or state laws allow it. Although this may surprise some people, most parents now keep babies who have died in their room for hours or even overnight without going to the morgue at all. Specific concerns and ways to keep the body cool are explained in the next section.

As many parents say, if this is all the time they will ever get with their child, they want to make the most of it. In fact, some parents make the decision that their babies will be "held their whole life" and coordinate with family members and staff to promote continuous holding time rather than keeping the baby in a bassinet or on the bed. You get to make this decision.

Some staff put the baby in warmed blankets. And some hospital staff keep the baby near the parents' room on the unit without bringing the baby to the morgue. If he is cared for in your room at the hospital or in your home, be aware that there will be slow deterioration, which is the natural progression. You will probably have a sense when it is time to give the baby up. Many parents have said they knew when it was time. Some fears parents have are almost irrational, but because they don't have experience with death, they feel real and make some sense to them. The baby won't fall apart, and he won't get as stiff as a board. If you have such questions, talk with the staff. Your questions and fears are felt by many; you are not the only one. Once you are more aware of what actually happens, you will be more comfortable with the idea of spending prolonged time with your baby.

BODY AND SKIN CARE AND GENERAL APPEARANCE

You might wonder about the condition of your baby's body, so some basics for you to consider follow. However, they do not ring true in every situation, and they should not stop you from being your baby's parent. If you had a two year old who had a horrible fall and was a bruised mess, would you love him less or not want to hold him? This is what parents do, looking beyond superficial appearances and following their parent heart or accepting appearances for what they are and loving their child anyway.

The early hours of holding your baby are reported as a most special time. Your baby will probably be warm from birth and then will begin to cool down. However, unless the baby is being held in the morgue, there is no reason for her to be ice cold. Many parents and hospital staff comment that the baby's appearance improves after a number of hours.

Many funeral directors suggest that in cool and moderate climates your child's body may be kept with you in a room without heating for up to thirty-six hours without any other precautions being taken, depending upon your state laws. Funeral directors and public health officials know these laws (though it always makes sense to ask for a copy).

Your baby's skin may appear darkened or reddened (like a severe sunburn) if he has been dead for a few days. The redness from blood near the surface lessens as the surface blood settles deeper inside the body. As a result, the skin color may lighten after a number of hours, becoming pale from lack of blood and oxygen. It will be gradual. Nothing happens suddenly, so you need not be shocked. There may be some skin tears, some normal leakage (use a tissue as you would if a living child's nose runs), or some spots where blood or fluids collect (sometimes described as similar to sunburn).

Your baby will become more fragile as time goes by. The baby's skin may start to peel and appear excessively dry. Because of the lack of oxygen and blood circulating in the body, the shape of your baby's face may change slightly. Usually no major changes occur in the first twenty-four to thirty-six hours. After that, changes occur slowly, not dramatically. Cooling your baby with ice packs, in a cooler, or with dry ice can slow the inevitable deterioration but can't stop it.

There are ways to keep your baby cool, which helps to slow deterioration, making it possible for you to keep the baby with you longer. A Cot Cooler is a cooling device placed underneath the baby. Some hospitals have them and may even let families borrow one to take their baby home for a day or two. Another method is using instant cold packs that can be used under and around a baby who is wrapped in blankets. They can be replaced as needed.

Your baby's body does stiffen slightly a few hours after the death, but that will not last. This idea may seem scary, but it need not be. The body will only be *somewhat firm* (probably not rigid) for a couple of hours and will then soften again. This is true for babies who are not placed in the morgue. Bodies coming from the morgue tend to be a bit more rigid for a little while due to the cold.

> I would never have believed how wonderful it could be to love up our baby while holding and rocking him for hours. Once we got over the fear, we just loved our time together as a family. Even our three year old got in on it and was better about it at first than we were. What a gift that time was! —Anonymous

> I told our nurse who helped us birth plan that I could not imagine holding my baby, let alone keeping her with us for two days (the example she gave was of a father who insisted the baby stay with them for two days). It sounded macabre! Then I had to eat my words. Once I met our beautiful daughter, I could not give her up. She stayed with us for three days while my wife recovered from a C-

section. The time was beautiful and way too short. Now our nurse has another story to tell, only instead of two, the record in her hospital is three days. —A daddy

NIGHTTIME

A few people have commented that they were unsure about being with their baby at night, while others cherished this peaceful, special time. It can be a lonely time and worries about what might happen to babies' bodies could be one concern. If you are more comfortable with the information we shared so far, you may be open to bedtime with your baby. Nothing more will happen during the night than during a normal day. This can be a very private, loving time, especially if it is your only night together.

Among other cultures (the Dutch, New Zealanders, the Amish, and some Native Americans, for example), babies and loved ones who died were cared for in their homes. This also happened in the United States prior to the 1930s or so. That means that parents kept their children in the parlor of the house and may have even slept with their children after death. Although you may not hear about this too often, it is happening all over the world and there is nothing odd about it.

When my sister, Hulda Mae, was stillborn, we played near her and my mother cared for her body in a loving way for a few days. I suppose it is possible she even slept with her. We kids got to meet her and even helped dig her grave. It was sad but so natural. —G. K.

TIPS AND ADVICE

- Ask your midwife, ob-gyn, or social worker any questions you might have about baby and baby's body. Do not be afraid to ask questions or hear the answers.
- Make sure that you get to do all that you wish to do with baby while you can. Unfortunately, this time will be much too short, and you will not be able to catch up on lost time.
- Invite as many people as you want to share this special time. This is your time, and those who are important to you should be there. Do

not force yourself either way. Be honest and be surrounded by only those you want and need.

- Seek peer support. Join a support group. If you've joined an online support group before baby's birth, you will be amazed at how supportive those groups can be after birth.
- Find an advocate or loss advisor. Women who have just given birth can be overwhelmed and may struggle at times with standing up for what they need. Get your advocate to speak on your behalf if need be and explain your wishes.

10

MEMORY CREATION

CREATING MEMORIES

Meeting your baby is a momentous time, one in which you will build many memories and shared experiences with your family. Memories are a key to healing in the long run, since they bring you close to your baby in the days and years ahead. Memories and mementos are the foundation for the healing; they serve as your reminders that you really did have a baby, that his little body was beautiful, that you are his mother or father, and that you have items that touched him or honored his little life. Memories will never take the place of your child, but they may provide a source of comfort in the years to come. Holding the outfit, touching the hair, feeling the footprints, and looking at pictures or videos help you to remember how you met and held your baby. Once you have delivered your baby, you should be able to have some private family time with him unless he is seriously ill and needs medical attention. You can continue to collect and make memories for the rest of your life.

SPENDING TIME WITH YOUR BABY

Hopefully, the hospital staff will accommodate most of your wishes. If not, call in your advocates to support you and work on your behalf as you negotiate the short but important time in the hospital. Care by advocates and advisors (who are often not hospital staff, but who work with you and the staff) is presently growing within many communities. And slowing things down—not rushing the birth—can give you some extra time to make plans and arrangements. You may find death doulas/ midwives, care companions, Baby Loss Doulas/Family Advisors, or perinatal loss specialists who can help you know your rights and guide you through the process of meeting and being with your baby. A few organizations and Facebook groups are listed in the Resources at the end of this book. If you have any questions that the doctor or nurses can't answer, ask a maternal/child manager at the hospital about parents' rights.

Memories and mementos are just as important if your baby lives for a while. The challenges your child faces may eventually result in her early death or the challenges may be lifelong and quite stressful. In either case, you'll long cherish these early moments, days, and weeks with your innocent, beautiful child, where you collected mementos, built memories, and shared time with your baby and others.

In this chapter you will find ideas to create, reinforce, and cherish your memories of your precious little one. Some will be easy to accomplish; others require planning. In the event that your birth was induced, you may still ask your midwife to take photos, and you should be able to see or hold your baby for a long time. Although short- and long-term memory making helps many families, it may not be easy for you right now. We highly recommend that you do it anyway, as you will never have another opportunity to make mementos or memories. You get this one moment in time.

PRIVATE TIME WITH YOUR BABY

While in the hospital, you can request a "do not disturb" sign for your door so that you can have some private time. You may need to reassure the staff that if you need anything or have any physical problems, you will call for a nurse. However, not everyone wishes to be in the hospital the entire time they are with their baby. They yearn for home and often are not told that they might have some time with baby at home. See chapter 11, "Saying Good-bye."

If you think it will be hard to look at mementos, you can put them away in a memory box and take them out when and if you are ready. Most parents report that they had no idea how important this special time was. They cherish the mementos and look back with confusion about how they could have thought that they wouldn't need such comfort-giving shared time and mementos.

Many parents tell of beautiful ways in which they interacted with their baby, including skin-to-skin contact, dancing with their baby to special music, taking their baby out into the sunshine, telling family stories, taking family photos, reading books, piercing ears, and painting fingernails. If you are fortunate to have some time at home with your baby, you may want to put her in the crib or bassinet in her room or take her to the swing set in the backyard. Open her eyes and examine your baby thoroughly; take lots and lots of pictures. Even if photos were taken at the hospital, you can never have too many pictures. Memories fade over time. You may even wish to play music and use certain scents such as baby lotion or powder or oils such as lavender or lemon. Smell is the most powerful and long-lasting sense.

Obviously, these suggestions are not a way to pretend your baby is alive, but to create that long-awaited bonding and loving time. It is also a time to begin to prepare for saying good-bye.

> When I walked into the bedroom, Stephanie was sitting on the bed holding Talina. I sat next to her, and we sat there just looking at Talina and soaking her in. It wasn't something I had planned to do, but it felt so natural and so beautiful. She was so perfect and I stroked her little brow and her tufts of hair. It was nice to be able to say all those usual things we say when someone has a baby like, "Doesn't she look like her brother!" And "Look at her little hands."
> —Narelle

Empty Arms by Sherokee Ilse and *When Hello Means Goodbye* by Pat Schweibert and Paul Kirk are two books that can be helpful if you have yet to deliver your baby or just delivered. They are full of wisdom from parents and staff who have lived through the experience of giving birth, meeting baby, and eventually saying good-bye. Why and how to create lifelong memories are explained, the pros and cons discussed, and specific ideas that can be easily adopted and used are shared. If you do not have these books, check with your clinic, doctor's office, or hospital, since they may have them available to aid parents during this important time.

This is also a good time to invite an advocate or companion to be with you who can help you to think about ways to enhance your time and improve the mementos that you will keep. She might also help find you resources (as might the hospital social worker or chaplain) for taking your baby home and for your emotional care. Visit the Resources at the end of this book to find information about where you can locate such caregivers.

> We wanted to create as many memories as possible with our daughter. We had my younger sister there to videotape the birth so that we could go back and relive every single moment of her precious life. This is one of my most cherished possessions. We also had many people taking pictures. We had approximately three rolls of film and a lot of digital camera cards full. I bought a foot-/handprint mold kit so that I could have her precious feet in my hands forever. I also created a scrapbook in her memory. It's filled with all of her pictures and beautiful sayings and poems. Last but not least, I have joined a memory box–painting program. We create boxes for families who lose their babies in hospital. —Anonymous

MEMORY CREATION THAT CAN BE PLANNED BEFORE OR AT BIRTH

Photos

Take a ton! It's better have too many than too few. Ask someone else to be in charge of the photos. You don't want to miss experiencing precious baby time. Take photos of your pregnancy, the birth, your baby in the special nursery, after death, and at the funeral. There are organizations such as Now I Lay Me Down to Sleep in the United States or Heartfelt in Australia with professional, volunteer photographers who may be able to take pictures of your baby and your family. Ask the staff about such a service.

Videos

A video of your baby and of your family meeting your baby shows movement and voices, which are comforting to have. Again, ask someone else to take them. Most smart phones have video options. Ask that all family and friends be included in the movies. This will be your best and only chance for such pictures, whether your baby lives or has already died. Get closeup shots of you, your partner, and children. Someday they may want proof or a reminder that they met their sibling. Take videos of the funeral or memorial service if you have one. You may not remember what happened and what was said due to shock and intense emotions. A video, or at least a recording, will be appreciated someday.

Pregnancy Reminders

Collect any hospital details, appointment cards, pregnancy test paperwork, ultrasound pictures, tummy pictures, train or parking stubs, wristbands, measuring tapes used to measure your baby, pamphlets, as well as other mementos that have meaning to you or that document details about your pregnancy or baby. You might even consider making a belly cast prior to birth; a beautiful three-dimensional memento.

Birth Reminders

Keep birth and death certificates, certificate of life, clothes your baby wore, a lock of hair, the umbilical cord clamp, nail clippings, blanket, items bought for the baby, newspaper headlines from that day, as well as any other details about the birth.

Handprints and Footprints

Staff often make footprints and handprints, including of babies who have died. Some funeral directors do plaster handprints and footprints for free or for a small fee. You can buy your own kit from some hobby and craft shops. You may also paint your daughter's nails and pierce her ears if you wish.

A Professional Hand-drawn Portrait

Consider a portrait. Experienced artists who work from photos will be able to soften the "marks" on your baby that you may want removed or highlight lovely features. Find them online or from support group referrals. Don't send original photos, which could get lost.

Sunrise or Sunset Pictures

An original photo taken on the day your child was born or died can help you remember that special day. You might not understand right now why this has meaning, but you might someday. A friend could do this for you.

A Diary

Write in a diary to keep memories fresh. Fill it with random thoughts, specific comments made, notes, poems, quotes, prayers, special photos, and so on. Write as often as you can or need to. Down the road, you will be grateful; it is common to forget many small details as time marches on. The fog of shock has a way of doing that.

Jewelry and Tattoos

It may be very nice to have a piece of jewelry that you can divide or separate, such as a set of earrings or a pendant, with one piece kept by mom (or dad, sibling, grandma, etc.) and the other with your child. The families who wore pendants, carried earrings, or had custom-made jewelry made speak highly of the sentimental value it brings. Pregnancy loss jewelry options are many and can be found all over the Internet. Tattoos are commonly used to remember babies who died. You'll find lots of options.

Funeral Arrangement Reminders

If you have a service, you may want to keep copies of the program, invoices, legal documents, pictures drawn for the baby by your other children or nieces or nephews, cards received, pressed flowers, a duplicate nameplate from the casket, a CD or list of the music played, as well as a list of what you placed in the casket and the guest list.

Celebrations

If you like, plan and celebrate joyful events, such as due dates, birthdays, and anniversaries of your little one. Some ideas for helping to celebrate your child over the years include annual picnics, visits to your child's grave, or special memorial activities such as planting trees or balloon or butterfly releases. Write your child's name with stones on the beach, build birdhouses, and even mention him in family newsletters.

One mother shared pictures of the picnic that was held at her daughter Amor's gravesite on the one-year anniversary of her death. They brought toys and activity bags for the children, food, music, and released balloons. An attitude of playfulness and fun was important to these parents, who miss their baby but wanted people to feel happy that she existed. Remembering her with fondness and fun was very important to them.

Another woman bought a small plant for her husband when their first child was stillborn. They tend the plant thirteen years later, taking clippings to start new plants and referring to them as "Gabriel's Garden." Her four other children help to care for the plants as well.

Holiday Donations

Many people find comfort in buying and donating presents for children who would have been the same age as their child during holidays such as Christmas. Or you could make and donate blankets, baby clothes, toys, and teddy bears for little ones who have died or are in the special care nursery.

Book Donation or Drive

Many pregnancy loss support groups and other family organizations have libraries filled with books and resources that are donated by parents in memory of their babies. This can be a special way to remember your child and make a difference in other parents' lives, too. Some parents run Facebook or social media book drives. They choose a favorite book to donate in bulk to area hospitals, then set a goal (say, one hundred copies) and ask family and friends to donate money to buy books.

Plant a tree

Plant a tree, bush, or flowers to commemorate your baby's life. You can also give a bush, flowers, or even bulbs to family and friends and ask them to plant them in their yards so that they will have nice memories throughout the years.

TIPS AND ADVICE

- Start thinking about your memory creation options. Ask others about what they've done and think about what you would like for yourself.
- Be mindful of the memory creation options that require planning. You may need to organize some ahead of time (for example, professional photo shoots or hand and foot molds).
- Save everything, even if you're unsure if you will want such mementos later. You can always discard what you don't want, but you won't be able to create these mementos later. Be open minded and think expansively.
- Some parents put the mementos and pictures away for a while. Others keep them close and visit them often. Find your way.

11

SAYING GOOD-BYE

Parents should never have to say good-bye to their child. All parents fully expect to die before their children, not the other way around. Yet here you are, saying good-bye to your baby who died despite your wishes, hopes, prayers, and even today's excellent medical expertise. As we have previously written, memories are what you will have as you go forward into the future. This is something you can do for your baby now. In the future, you won't have birthday parties full of children, you won't go to his first dance or prom, and sadly, there won't be a wedding. What you can do is give your child a special good-bye ceremony.

The process begins with spending time saying good-bye to your child's physical body—in the hospital, at home if you choose, or at the funeral home prior to and during the ceremony if you have one. You may not be familiar with how to do this, and you wouldn't want to do it if you had a choice. But if you make this time special for you, your other children, and your family and community, you will find some comfort and eventual peace.

It's difficult to process the practical aspects of planning rituals and handling the disposition of your child's body when you are overwrought with emotions. If you did some preplanning in your birth plan, this may be a bit easier, though it still will be a painful process. You may also have been reluctant to make such plans because you were not ready to think about your baby's death or you did not believe your baby would really die. In any case, you will now need to make those decisions and plan a special good-bye. You may be Jewish and expect to sit Shiva,

Muslim and have less than twenty-four hours to bury your baby, or a Christian with varying traditions. Maybe you don't have a particular religion and must give thought to your understanding of death and what type of burial or cremation you prefer. We leave those specifics to you. Some ideas in this chapter may inspire you as you make your own decisions according to your own beliefs and wishes.

Many experts, grief specialists, and family members encourage spending time with your child as a natural next step after death. It is both the hello time and too quickly the good-bye time, especially for new parents who have waited for so long to meet their child. Finally seeing and holding the baby makes her real and gives you memories for the future. It also allows others to see her as her own person, not just a belly bump. However, that is not the case with some families. If you are adamant that you prefer not to—or feel unable to—spend much time with your baby, that is okay, too. Each person must follow his or her own judgment. After all, you are the parents of this child and have the right to decide.

TRANSITION FROM HOSPITAL TO HOME, FUNERAL HOME, OR CREMATORIUM

Previously, we wrote of spending all the time you can with your baby at the hospital and at the funeral home. You may wish to remain with your baby until she is given to the funeral director or is cremated. In most states and countries, parents are responsible for making decisions about burial and cremation if the baby is older than twenty weeks. Practices vary for babies less than twenty weeks. Some parents now ask to hand the baby over to the funeral director. This can be done in the hospital room rather than the morgue. It is another way to allow you to care for your own child. Families who have checked out of the hospital have asked nurses to hold their babies until the funeral directors arrive. Parents felt reassured that their baby was not alone but held and loved throughout the process. A family member or advocate may be able to help work out these details, if you do not wish to get involved in these discussions or can't bring yourself to talk about your baby's burial or cremation. Hopefully, you will clear up such details prior to the birth. There are parents who prefer that their babies be picked up at the morgue by the funeral director. Be aware that though you may be responsible for the burial or cremation of your baby, there is no requirement for a funeral service. Unlike many families who have a sudden death, you have some time to work through these details. *Planning a Precious Goodbye*, by Sherokee Ilse and Susan Erling Martinez, and *When a Child Dies: A Resource for Families*, by Trina Charles and Heidi Ciepielinski, offer specific assistance in planning services including poems, songs, readings, types of service ideas, and more.

Of course, saying good-bye to your child in the physical sense will never be easy under any circumstances. Clearly, only you will determine what is best in your own situation. Like every other parent, when you look back, you inevitably will think of things you wish you had done. As mommy or daddy, you will crave a lifetime with your child; sadly, that has been taken from you.

Some religions require burial or cremation within a tight time frame, even as quickly as twenty-four hours. If this is the case, your options for time together in the hospital may be limited. You will need to make the most of the time you have. Spend your time with your baby alone, as a couple, and with family if you can. Examine your baby fully and say your physical good-byes. As hard as this will be at the time, you will be grateful you had such special time. Many funeral directors are sensitive to the death of a child, especially a newborn; you may find that they are very open to allowing you to come to the funeral home and spend time dressing and holding your baby. In fact, many have rocking chairs that can be used for this and private rooms for dressing. If they are experienced with babies' deaths and if they are open to parent involvement, you may be encouraged to bring your other children with you. Although you may be reluctant, we can reassure you that if you want to do this and have an appropriate, gentle attitude about it, you may find this to be a special time. Many parents say that the children usually handle it better than the adults. Again, after fair consideration and discussion with others who may have been through this, you may conclude this is not for you. Do not worry. You'll do your best at making the best decisions you can.

TRANSPORTING YOUR BABY

Transporting your baby to the funeral home, the crematorium, the cemetery, or even to your home for a short time with the proper paperwork and support may be an option. This could be a helpful step in the good-bye process for you. You might wish to request a funeral director or another designated family member (if allowed) to bring your beloved baby to his final resting place.

In order to do this, you will need to learn how to transport his body, if permitted by your laws. A container such as a basket or even a car seat can be used. You may want ice packs in the bottom to help cool your baby. Think of what you would do if your baby were alive—have a blanket and hat ready. Also, ask the hospital to provide you with a form or a letter that states that you are parents transporting your baby who has already died. On the off chance that you are stopped by the police for some reason or are in a minor accident, you will not want the authorities to be suspicious of you.

Maybe you prefer the funeral director to drive your baby in his car and you want to ride along to stay close to your baby. Have a conversation about such options prior to a final decision. If home is the destination for a few hours or a day, another option is to have the funeral director drive your baby from the hospital to your home. Discuss your options with the funeral director, who can inform you about the laws and your rights.

BRINGING YOUR BABY HOME

More and more parents wonder about bringing their babies home after death. Parenting opportunities at home, combined with the privacy and security aspects, are tempting. Instead of only hospital memories, parents can have their baby beside them in bed, in the crib, in an infant seat, and rock the baby, which will be wonderful memories for later. If they choose to have an open house or small celebration of life at home, it can save money and be more personal. Not all states allow family home care after death, but most do. (Only nine states have laws prohibiting it. *Final Rights*, a book and a website, explains this further and lists those states.) Too many hospitals prohibit this choice despite the state laws that allow it. So this may or may not actually be an option for you.

If you would like to take your baby home for a short period, learn if there will be barriers. The sooner you look into it, the better. This may be a unique thought for you and you might feel uncomfortable about it, which makes sense if you haven't had experience with it. Some Native Americans and communities like the Amish do this consistently. And some countries like New Zealand and Holland also expect most families to take their loved ones home for post-death care. In fact, that was the way death was handled a century ago in the United States. Post-death care at home is slowly returning and will likely continue to grow as a viable option.

However, don't feel pressure to do this if you are uncomfortable with the idea. If, however, it interests you, ask hospital professionals or a funeral director about the laws (not the common practice, but the law). Be aware that hospital staff may not yet be comfortable with this idea, but in the end, remember whose baby it is and who should have the right within the law and within the confines of what is healthiest for you and your family. Do what seems right for you and your family. A funeral director, death midwives, loss family advisors, care companions, or other advocates know how to help. Your home funeral guide or midwife and the website www.BringYourBabyHome.com can help inform you about this practice and why it is being revived in our modern culture.

Some worry that parents will never want to let their children go if they take them home. This is rarely true. Parents have said that because they had precious time with their babies in a comfortable, homey environment, it was actually easier to let go, because they saw subtle physical changes occur in their babies' bodies. This helped them to know when it was time to let go. Most parents lament that there was not enough time and opportunity to be with their baby to do things like dressing and undressing or bathing the baby using their own bathtub and soap or spending time with the baby in her room, rocking, singing, and storytelling. You will never feel you had enough time, but you will know when to let go.

Learn about other people's experiences to determine if it is a positive alternative for your family. For some parents of young children, the option of taking a baby home is appealing. The peaceful, safe place they know as home can be a calm and secure haven during this unbelievable time. For older siblings, being with their baby sister or brother at home can be very special as they touch, hold, ask questions, even play while their baby sister or brother is nearby. Children are rarely familiar with or comfortable in hospitals, and sometimes there are rules limiting the amount of time children can stay. That makes it more complicated to accomplish what you wish to as a family. Most children are less uptight about death than adults, which can turn time at home into a special, memorable experience. Don't be afraid if there are tears and sadness, there will also be smiles and probably even levity as you explore the baby and spend time together as a family.

CHOOSING NOT TO TAKE BABY HOME

Remember, there is nothing wrong with *not* bringing your baby home. Perhaps it will be too difficult. Perhaps it is not allowed. Perhaps you believe it will make separating later even harder. Whatever you decide is what will work best for you. Your choice of how you will remember and where you will care for your baby—or not—is your choice. Just remember, you don't know what you have never been prepared for, so talk with others who have been there and read books or websites of others who have seen the long-term consequences of their decisions.

> I was adamant that I did not want to see our baby [other than] from across the room and that we would not spend time with her. She was dead and probably stiff and might smell—the whole thing sounded disgusting. The staff tried to change my mind, but I held strong. About six months later when I woke up and realized I had missed my opportunity to rock and discover my little girl, I was truly upset. I realize I was scared and in shock. Not a good time to make such decisions. And I learned later that all my worries were pretty unfounded. Why didn't I listen? —A mom

> I am fine with my decision to hold my baby for only a few minutes, take a few pictures, and move on. It all seemed surreal and I just wanted to go home. We have come to accept that decision and don't hold too much guilt about it. —A mom

RITUALS

No parent ever expects to have to plan a funeral, good-bye ceremony, celebration of life, or cremation for a newborn. It goes against nature and the plans you have made for a life with your child. Chances are, you have not faced too many deaths yet. Like most people of childbearing age, making plans for your own funeral and burial is not something you have done. Facing your own mortality at such a young age also seems unnatural.

You may worry about the cost and hate the idea of having to now make plans to bury or cremate your child. If you can agree on a ceme- tery and a plan for yourselves, it will be easier to make a decision for your baby. If not, you will want to explore ideas such as the possibility (and cost) of someday moving the casket or perhaps you might choose cremation since you can retain the ashes and keep them with you wherever you go.

You may feel as if you are in deep shock and a bit robotic as you go through the motions while still in a zombie-like fog. For this reason, we (and other parents) encourage you to make sure that someone video- tapes the service for later viewing and even to share with any young siblings or subsequent children someday.

Some parents choose not to have a funeral for their child but have a private graveside service or a ceremony at a later time. You may decide to have your baby cremated, keeping the ashes in a special place in your home or scattering them in a special place. It is up to you. The books mentioned earlier and other resources can help you gather music, poems, and appropriate readings. You will even find ideas about how and why to write an obituary.

> This is something I am glad we had the courage to do and talk about while we were still expecting the baby. We didn't want to be nega- tive, but there was a 60 percent chance we would have to organize a funeral. Talking about this while you are still carrying your baby is one of the most horrible feelings a parent can go through, but I am glad we did. We found a song to play at the funeral, "Somewhere over the Rainbow" by Eva Cassidy. The funeral organizing, the day or two after Gabby passed, was so hazy and surreal that I am glad we had found her special song beforehand. —Anonymous

CHOOSING A FUNERAL DIRECTOR

Funeral directors are an important resource if you want help with the funeral. They can give advice about obituaries, casket options, music, flowers, balloons, and readings. Someone should interview the director to ensure that she or he has experience with babies' funerals. Also ask about ways that they can make it special, such as having a rocking chair so that you can rock baby, inviting family to help dress baby before the service, and involving your other children. Make sure you feel comfortable with the answers and that you feel good about entrusting your baby into her or his care. If not, find another. Trust your instinct here. This is the only funeral ritual or celebration you will have for your child in the physical sense. You want it to be as perfect as possible while minimizing regrets.

THE SERVICE

Make this as special as you can. Although it is a farewell for your child, it can also be a celebration of his life on Earth. You may hear ideas or suggestions from family and close friends or you may wish to invite them to give you ideas. As part of your close circle and community, they are connected and love you and your baby. Work to give serious consideration to their ideas, while making it what *you* want it to be—you get the final say; this is your baby.

Whether you have the service at a funeral home, your chosen religious meeting place, the interfaith chapel at the hospital, or your own home, you may have the choice of a closed or open casket (so that your baby can be seen one last time, especially by those who may not have met him). You may wish to include toys, flowers, balloons, photos, decorations made by family prior to or as a part of the service, beautiful music, poems, or whatever moves you.

Find out if there are people who want to participate in some way in your special good-bye. Someone may want to sing, make the casket, sew or knit the burial outfit or blanket, or donate flowers from their garden. Someone may even wish to officiate. There is so little that others will be able to do for your child, so now may be the time to extend the invitation. Often fathers have a need to do something, so be sure you have a conversation before rather than afterward, when it is too late.

There are helpful resources for saying good-bye listed at the back of this book, such as HeavensGain.com, where you can find beautiful urns and caskets. There are a few good booklets to help you to plan a service, which offer poetry, lists of songs, small sample readings, advice about what to write in an obituary, and more. There are even some organizations that may be able to help pay a portion of the cost of the funeral or headstone.

BURIAL OR CREMATION

If you cremate your baby, you can keep her with you in a special urn, which allows you to feel close to her. You can bring her with you if you move and you can even have her buried with you one day. Some of the ashes can be put inside a locket or even a teddy bear. Build-a-Bear Workshop is one company that offers this option and there are others.

If you decide to bury your child, you will have a place to visit as a family or alone. It might comfort your children, and if you move away someday, you may be able to move the casket (if it was kept inside a vault or strongbox that won't deteriorate) to be reburied at a different cemetery. If you think this might happen, let the funeral director and cemetery manager know so that the proper procedures are followed that will make it possible down the road.

> Life, as I am coming to find out, throws you for a loop sometimes and no matter what you plan for, it might not always work out. So say something happens, like a job transfer or we decide to retire far away, I don't want to be separated from where my baby is buried. But what if, fifty years from now, my husband and I no longer live here and we go forward with our own burial plots, can we move the baby to take him with us at that time? And if not, then do we buy our plots now where the baby is? I mean, the cemetery where he will be is very small. I doubt in fifty years there will space for us. So does that force us to buy our burial plots now to ensure we are never separated? —Toni-Marie

ADDITIONAL CONSIDERATIONS

Once you have organized the bulk of the service, you may wish to give other ideas and options some thought. With burials, the casket is rarely considered an option, but its size or shape may be. For example, you may decide to pick a casket of a particular size if you want enough room to place toys or other items in it. Influenced by children in your family, perhaps you want to put special stickers or decorations on the casket. Some families have had their living children draw on the casket, making their baby's precious vessel unique and full of memories.

Press notices and obituaries can be a tangible reminder to keep. The funeral director can help with this if you need it. Releasing doves or butterflies can be a lovely and uplifting way to conclude your child's service. A portrait or sketch of the baby by a professional artist could also be a wonderful reminder. Keep a guest book to capture names and messages. Some funeral directors do handprint and footprint molds; ask about this if it isn't offered. Some funeral homes in the United States bake cookies or a cake for a pre- or post-service gathering. One mortuary even offers to make bears using the loved one's clothing, though this usually occurs in the ensuing months, not necessarily at the time of the funeral. Perhaps this is an idea for a family seamstress who wants to contribute to the service in some way, or you could save some of the clothing, find a pattern online, and make your own bear or other keepsake someday. Use your imagination and make this experience as special as you can.

TIPS AND ADVICE

- Ask others for advice and help. Being in a fog impacts clarity of thought. Stephanie chose her daughter's burial plot while pregnant. Only months after the funeral, she realized that the plot she chose was crowded amid many other plots. Had she been thinking more clearly at that time, she would have chosen a corner plot or a garden bed to lay her daughter to rest.
- Ask for advice from support group members or online friends in the baby loss community. What worked for them? What didn't?

- Do not rush. Although you might be pressured to make decisions on the spot, the truth is that you probably have at least a few days or weeks (or months, if you're still pregnant) to decide. Take the time to make the *right* decision for you.
- Do not be afraid to ask questions. Unless you ask, you will never know what is or isn't an option. This is an important ritual and you deserve for it to be the best.

II

The Journey of Ending the Pregnancy

We are so sorry that your baby has been diagnosed with difficulties and that you are here now. Depending on when you find this book, you may feel as though you were—and still are—in a deep, dark place enveloped in fog. Shock helps insulate you from reality. But it is also an eerie place to be, where sometimes you may not know who you are and how you got here. You may feel haunted, defenseless, and exposed. Your protective bubble has burst and you are now vulnerable to even more pain. "Why me?" you may ask. How could this have happened, shattering your future, your hopes, and your dreams?

It isn't fair. You were parents heading toward a beautiful life. Things changed, and amidst deep shock and disbelief, you were given unexpected information and then asked to make a decision you may never have foreseen. You were asked to play God and decide whether your pregnancy would continue or end, whether your child would die sooner or later. Surely this is an unexpected path. You thought that you had things under control and now you realize that you have little control at all. You love your baby and would never, ever hurt him. Yet you had to make a horrific decision—to choose between allowing your baby to suffer and likely be in pain or putting an end to that suffering sooner. Or maybe mom's life was endangered and there really was no choice; it was made for you. All this has been done through love, and you will review it in your mind for a long time. Your heart will hurt much longer.

Love is like that. We are never ready to let our sweet children go. Never.

Maybe you were fortunate to have caregivers who offered you the option of making a birth plan or having a birth vision to guide your delivery or your dilation and curettage or dilation and evacuation procedures and to meet your baby. Although meeting baby in this situation is only a few decades old, it continues to grow as a choice made by loving parents. If you did not have this opportunity but wish you had, write a letter or call someone at the clinic or hospital where you gave birth and suggest that mothers (and fathers) in your situation be offered this option to reduce fear and to help families plan for the birth and beyond. This doesn't make it better for you, but it may feel good to pay it forward.

> We chose to suffer a lifetime of pain to spare you—Carter William George—from one second of it. —Danielle Townsend

As you look back on the last few hours, days, or more, you probably realize that the dreams you held for your baby and your family's future did not include this. You are not alone. Countless parents find themselves in this situation. Since others have come before you, there are messages and suggestions from them about how to go forward. They—and we—want you to know that there is love and support here for you to aid in this unchartered journey. Here, experienced navigators offer guidance as you make your way through the wreckage following the unexpected bomb that shattered your life. Living through this requires information, support, and love. Who knows, but maybe someday you will be one of those who assist and support other parents in this situation.

You may wonder where you go next and how you will ever survive. Whether your decision was based on religious or spiritual grounds, moral or ethical considerations, fear for mom's health, family pressure, concerns that your baby would suffer, personal needs and fears, or financial or health reasons, among others, you are here now. Hopefully, as you answered that incomprehensible question about what you were going to do, you made the decision that you can live with the best. The one that will haunt you the least. The one that seems the least difficult for you, though, of course, is never easy.

Termination is often talked about as a "choice"—we make a choice to end the pregnancy at that time. But what about when that choice does not feel like a choice, or when that choice (although potentially a better option for all involved) feels like you are committing the ultimate offense against life? Often this is where women are left without appropriate support in working their way through a moral minefield. —Carolyn, *Holding On & Letting Go*

We describe the decision-making time like being stuck at the top of a high mountain; there are two ways down, one was to jump off the steep side and the other was to roll down the rocky side. In both cases, we knew we might not be alive by the time we got to the bottom. There is no easy or less painful choice, really. —A dad

The rest of the story is now our life! How do we live with ourselves and in our community knowing we jumped and gave our baby an easier way out of the suffering? The only answer we have come to is—one day at a time and one step at a time. We work hard not to be too hard on ourselves (well, most of the time, that is) and we no longer judge people for anything, because we know how much it hurts to feel the judgment of others. No one can feel worse about this than us. —A mom

As you may have read earlier in this book, we assume that most people who have ended their pregnancies have already done so by the time they pick up this book. Once a fatal diagnosis is delivered, there is usually a tight window for action and not much time to really prepare well for the birth and meeting your baby, which is then quickly followed by the good-byes. Consequently, we pick up from there, offering reality and hope for living beyond the decision you made and the birth of your baby. We cover many aspects in both parts II and III that we hope will help you to navigate the rocky path ahead. However, if you did get this book early enough, you may find some help in part I regarding birth, meeting your baby, memory making, and saying good-bye.

12

LIVING BEYOND THE DECISION

LOSS OF YOUR DREAMS

Once you are home after the procedure that rocked your world, you are probably still numb and in shock. Who wouldn't be? This is not your dream, not your plan. When you learned your baby had a life-limiting diagnosis, the solid ground you stood on became full of crevices and canyons, as deep and wide as the Grand Canyon itself. There was no safe ground anymore and your sense of security and safety was lost. How can parents be asked to consider ending their beloved child's life when their very goal has been to give life and protect it? If mom's life was in danger, you may be even more deeply in shock, realizing that both of you could have died. No matter how you got here, now you are forced to deal with it. By now, you have probably buried or cremated your child. You wonder what to do next. The darkness encompasses you and nothing much makes sense anymore.

> That night our minds raced, our hearts broke, and we made that choice. . . . We decided we wanted to stop his suffering and meet him. As we walked into that hospital that day, my life changed forever. —Danielle

GOOD DAYS AND BAD DAYS

As you struggle to go forward, you will have good days and you will have bad days. Expect them both. There are any number of issues that may rumble around in your mind. Numb and still in shock, you may have few coherent thoughts. This is normal and yet it is not. You may find it hard to believe that you once had a sane, planned, happy life. Now you may be wandering the ruins of this life you don't even recognize. There is much work to do and much to learn as you struggle on the present course.

> After getting the news that the test was positive, the news was not good. . . . Over the next few days we blocked the world out. We spent every waking hour together talking about the options. I cried so much. Even now, I cry. I felt so sad. Sad for us, sad for the baby, sad for our family. . . . She was a baby. One minute I felt that the only ethical option was to terminate the pregnancy. The next minute I felt ripped up inside that I could even consider killing my baby. Those words are so harsh [that] they still make me wince. But they are truthful. We found it incredibly difficult to decide . . . though we did decide to terminate in the end. —Margaret, *Holding On & Letting Go*

COMMON FEARS AND CONCERNS

What do you say to others about your little one? Maybe you are in the throes of the darkness of grief and mourning. You may be haunted by the induction and the hospital time and need to work through those feelings and review what happened. Hopefully, you were encouraged to meet your baby and make some memories to cherish over time. You are still this child's parent and you will need to discover how to keep your baby close, though she is not physically in your arms. Returning to work is an issue if you work outside the home. If you have a partner, you'll need to figure out the plan soon. This topic is explored further in chapter 21, "Workplace Issues."

There are many things to think about and you may have many questions and fears.

- What do you say to others?
- Did you say good-bye to your sweet baby in a meaningful way?
- Have you made the right decision?
- Do you have the courage and strength to go forward?
- What will you tell friends and family who knew that you were expecting?
- Will you feel guilty, and if so, how will you deal with that?
- Is forgiveness a component of healing?
- Will others blame you?
- Are you the only one who has been through such a traumatic pregnancy?
- How do you find others who "get it"?
- What if you have regrets?
- What resources might you need?

BEING THE PARENT

You are, and always will be, this child's parent. How you spent time with your baby after birth has now become a memory. Memories are a key to healing over time, so cherish everything you have and make more memories over time. You were pregnant and now are not. The physical changes that mom feels are real. So are the emotional ones that you both experience, though only mom experiences hormonal changes. Regardless of how the pregnancy ended, that time and what happened will be there waiting to be dealt with. There is no way to avoid pain, because when you love someone and he or she dies—no matter when—it will always hurt and it will always be difficult. But if you go forward with confidence that you are not alone and that you can survive and be strong again, you will have a better chance of getting there.

Build a foundation of love and memories that can provide comfort in the dark days ahead. You are your child's parent and what was done was done out of pure love. Keep being that parent in the days ahead, and keep your love boldly alive. You are still a parent whose baby died. No one can take that away. The memories of your pregnancy journey will become sweet memories once again if you allow that to happen. Your love will always be there. Your child knew only your love and a perfect life inside you, mom. Now you are left to go forward and carry on the legacy of someone special who lives on through you. Focus on going forward, since you can't change the past. If you feel that you need forgiveness, seek it from your child, God, your partner, and yourself. Eventually, when you find some acceptance, you may find some peace on your own timetable, or God's, if you are a spiritual person. Include your child in family gatherings (perhaps light a candle during holidays or special days). Speak of your child openly; it may not be easy in the beginning but it will come more naturally the more you do it. Buy presents and toys for others in the name of your child, celebrate his birthdays, and tell his story. You have this right as his mother and father. Feel the pride and love that is within your heart. And if you can't do these things now, that's okay. Trust your judgment that you will know what you need to do when you get there.

Face your feelings about how you were told and how you were treated. You may hold hard feelings about how you were given the news or the advice your doctor or nurse offered. You might feel that you were treated poorly or were not supported as well as you deserved. You may even have felt pressure to have a dilation and curettage (D&C) or dilation and evacuation (D&E) procedure rather than an induction, where you might have had a whole baby to see. It is also possible that you feel you were given great care and are grateful to everyone and for what they did for you.

Cherish your memories and work to create more over time. Rituals, mementos, and memories of the time you had with your baby are to be held dear. Keep them in your memory box and your heart. Perhaps you could hold a celebration of her life at a later point or release doves at a park or cemetery in her honor. You might wish to look online for the many baby items made as keepsakes for parents like you. There are any number of jewelry items, some of which could hold ashes or might have your baby's handprint or footprint on the piece. Cherish these keepsakes and memories and share them with others as you see fit. Much peace and comfort can result over time. These are your connections to your baby and the time you held her close within.

Guilt is common, natural, and should be allowed, as long as it does not overwhelm you and your life. Not feeling guilt is okay, too. Mom, if your life was saved by ending your pregnancy, you may still be reeling from the guilt and the suddenness of it all. Quite a few mothers say that they would have gladly given their lives if their babies could have lived.

However, dad, your other children, and your family probably feel the opposite. Though they would never wish for your child to die, they cannot fathom the thought of you dying. You may never be on the same page about this, so find others, sisters in sorrow and love. You love your baby more than life. Motherhood is like that, so it is understandable that you would dive in to save your drowning child, even it meant that you might drown. But this will be hard for your partner to imagine.

> As every minute passed, I drew closer to death. Within a few minutes of hearing the doctor's words, "It's either one of you (meaning me) or both of you," I nodded in agreement for an induction . . . at nineteen weeks my son could not survive. By agreeing to an early induction, I became a mother who had to step aside and allow harm to come upon my child. At that exact moment, I lost a piece of myself.
> —Jennifer Ross, *Isaiah's Story*

Acknowledge the normalcy of grieving for someone you love and learn to mourn well.

If you could "get over" the loss of a family member—or in this case, your baby—easily, then what is the value and importance they held in your life? Deep love and high hopes equal deep loss and dreams dashed. This only makes sense. Once you understand why it makes sense and that this will be a painful, long process—because he or she was, and still is, important and well-loved by you—you may be able to let your feelings flow. Better that than holding them inside. In order to heal, which is not about forgetting or recovering, you'll need to do the hard work of mourning well. Learn more about how to grieve and mourn (the outward expression of your feelings) in chapter 23, "Grief and Healing." Also read books about grief and healing.

OTHER THINGS TO CONSIDER

You may find that you feel "out of it." It may be hard to get out of bed, to make meals, to go back to work, to tend the yard, to interact with others, and to think and make rational decisions. You will start to see a pattern, and around the time you get used to it, things will change. For example, in the early days, you may not want to leave the bedroom or the house, and you might discourage (or encourage) visitors. Eating might seem unimportant and you may not pay much attention to your children. If this is the case, do ask your parents or another close relative to move in, to visit often, or even to take the children for a few hours each day. Explain what is happening to your children so that they do not feel abandoned. You could say you feel so sick that you can't get out of bed and need your rest. Explain that it is hard to make meals or to take care of the house and that this won't last forever (trust us, it won't last). Perhaps you need someone to take care of you, too. This is understandable. Your world has shattered and the landscape is in ruins.

After a while, you may be able to get out of bed for coffee or have enough energy to make a bakery or deli run. But still you might feel tired and washed out—you've just had a medical procedure, a delivery, so this is normal on both a physical and an emotional level. It is hard to find energy when in a state of crisis and sadness. You may have moments when you can accomplish something and moments when you feel useless. Some parents go back to work part time or take a longer leave if needed. You'll find that you lose things easily and can't remember why you went from one room to another. All of this is very typical.

Anger may be hard to handle, especially for many women. Men come to anger more easily and may look for an outlet. There are many reasons for anger now, as it is a vital part of mourning for many. You mourn for your lovely pregnancy that went awry and for your precious little one. You can't believe how harsh the world has suddenly become. You notice that others go on with life as though nothing happened. In addition, you may be angry with hospital staff, strangers, coworkers, family members, or God. Some say it is better to be angry with someone other than your partner or close family members, since you don't have to live with him or her. If it makes you feel better, put your feelings about the hospital or the hospital staff on paper. Then either tear it up (which might make you feel better) or send it to them if not too harsh. They need to know what helped and what did not help so that they can improve their care and it also might be therapeutic for you.

> I do not remember feeling anger in the year following our son's stillbirth. I focused on grieving and helping others. Near the end of the first year, I decided to go for a massage. While working on my back, the therapist asked, "Are you angry about something significant?" Out of the blue, I burst into tears and couldn't stop. I told her what had happened—that our son had died. I agreed that, indeed, I

was very angry. But I had not allowed myself to acknowledge it at all! Anger is not something to hold onto if we want to be healthy. I wish I knew better how to express it and I am thankful that this massage therapist was so aware and dared to ask me. —Sherokee

WORDS THAT HURT

You also may have been hurt or upset by words that medical professionals or others used when talking with you. Some of those words or phrases may be "incompatible with life," "termination," "interruption," "fetus," "late-term abortion," "medical abortion," "kill the baby," or "products of conception." These words were not chosen to intentionally hurt you; many of them are commonly used medical phrases. Despite protests of many parents, medical jargon is not easy to change. In this book, the words used are "ending the pregnancy," "termination," or "interruption." No harm or judgment is intended. You may not prefer such words; we understand. It is hard to meet everyone's needs. Hopefully, you are able to move beyond that as you continue to read and as you interact with others who struggle with words to describe what has happened. The fact remains, you don't have to adopt or use those words. Tell others what you prefer when speaking about your child. Say the words "daughter" or "son" to show personhood. Eventually, others will pick up on your language and probably use it also—at least within your community, even if the medical professionals do not.

Hopefully, you were treated like the mother (and father) you are, not a medical patient who went in for a "procedure." You deserved chances to see your baby, collect mementos, and create special memories. This was all the time you had with your baby in a physical sense. If you did not get this gentle, loving, care, we are sorry if you feel that you missed out. Although you cannot change the past, you can lodge a complaint, write a letter, or ask for a meeting someday when you are ready. The administration and the staff on the surgery or labor and delivery units deserve to know the implications of their care. If they did things well, tell them that as well.

In the days ahead you will have mixed emotions; let them come. Each has a place in your heart and your journey. This is your baby's story, your family's story. When you find yourself in need of support, check out the many national and regional resources that may offer you some advice, comfort, and a sense of community. Find books and other resources that speak to you in a language of love and parenthood that you will understand.

TIPS AND ADVICE

- Make sure to take your time to review and process your decision and its implications in your life. You'll need to make peace with yourself, one another, and maybe others, including your baby.
- You have made the *better* decision for you and your baby; no one should try to deny or take this away from you.
- Access supportive professionals. Find someone who accepts your decision and compassionately supports you.
- Keep talking to people you trust—a friend, relative, or professional about your feelings and fears.
- Join a support group or find others in the same situation. Warm, nonjudgmental peer support is invaluable.
- Be kind to yourself. This is a traumatic time. You may feel a sense of guilt about having your baby early. Remind yourself that those emotions are normal, including guilt. Don't let it fester inside of you. Share it with others who understand, write about it, pray about it, and seek forgiveness if you feel it is right. Recognize that guilt is a common feeling that can't easily be erased, but you can cope with it and prevent it from ruining your life.
- Be sure to get follow-up medical care and mental health care if needed.
- Be the parent you are. Since getting the confirmation that you were pregnant, you have been a mommy or a daddy. Now that your child has died, you continue to hold that title, and, in fact, you have suffered the ultimate in parenthood, burying your child whom you loved dearly. Keep parenting and loving your son or daughter. You'll know how or seek advice from others who do.

13

REGRETS AND GUILT

Although we have dealt with regret and guilt in a more general manner in the introduction, we are aware that this topic is a burden for many parents, so we revisit it here with specific regard to the decision to induce or terminate your pregnancy. There is little in life as intense and difficult as having a baby die, especially in this way.

QUESTIONING YOUR DECISION

No matter which choice parents make, feelings of regrets and guilt are typical. Questioning whether this was the right decision may bubble forth for you, or you may be secure that this is what needed to be done. You would never have chosen this, and it didn't feel like a choice at all. Your baby was precious and wanted, but after learning of the problems, everything changed.

The lack of time prior to being pressed for a decision may add to your doubts about whether you made the right one. It is understandable. This was a life-and-death decision that has incredible implications for you, your baby, and your family. And when you are in shock but asked to make life-altering decisions, often within a few days, it can be difficult to find clarity or to benefit from the wisdom of others who have been in such situations.

You will need to work through it in your mind and heart. For many, this will take much work. Don't assume you must—or can—do this by yourself. Counseling and lots of support may help in the healing process. However, in your place of vulnerability, get referrals for therapists who have some understanding and experience with this issue. You do not need to be hurt further by well-meaning counselors who don't have training and experience with such families as yours.

> My husband and I wonder constantly, did we make the right decision? Could our child have been a miracle baby who defied the doctor's predictions? How do we live with ourselves for the rest of our days knowing that the question remains unanswered? What if he could have been healthy and lived? —A mom and dad

> It was hell making a decision. No parent should ever have to do this. But we did. And now we live without regrets, knowing that it was the best we could do. Our child is at peace, though we miss her terribly. —Parents of a child with trisomy 13

You may worry that not only do you feel upset, but others may not understand your decision and the parental pressures you faced. Now you face family, community, and societal opinions. All this can add to the stress and emotional weight you carry.

THE STIGMA OF THE WORD "ABORTION"

Regrets and guilt are a human condition for virtually all people. Adding to that, there is social stigma surrounding this decision. The word "abortion" suggests different thoughts and opinions for different people. For you, under your circumstances, it may not seem like the right word at all. This colors things for you. You may not want to say "abortion" when you are asked what happened to your baby. Telling your family and children isn't easy. Making sense of it in your heart is also something you must endure.

> It took me years to get beyond daily guilt. There was a lot of repeating to myself, "there was nothing that I could do." I take his presence in daily. Though I cannot see him . . . I feel him. It's been a lot of faith walking along the journey. —Jennifer

You may repeat and relive questions like, Why did we have to choose? Why did we have to have that procedure? Why is it called an abortion? Why did we have to have it in a place where others were ending their unwanted pregnancies? Why didn't we spend more time with our baby or invite our family to see her? So much about this situation seems unfair and it leads to stress and other feelings that weigh on your heart.

Perhaps you don't believe in abortion or have firm religious beliefs prohibiting it and yet you felt compelled to take this route. Those long-held beliefs, which may also be held within your family, do not go away easily or at all. You'll need to reconcile them someday. We'll talk about forgiveness and grace later, which might help when you are ready. Your rabbi, minister, priest, or other religious leader might help.

Perhaps you had to have the procedure in a facility that does abortions of unwanted babies. This can cause even more heartache. It is the ultimate slap in the face. Some parents report little genuine support and sensitivity during this time. Maybe you were upset and uncomfortable sitting near other women about to abort. It shouldn't have been like that for you, and the guilt may pile on, since you never expected to be in such a position at such a place. Whether you are pro-life or pro-choice, this is no longer simply a philosophy or a topic for debate; it is a personal trauma that affects *you*. You may look at the whole issue differently now.

REGRETS

If you birthed your baby but were not provided with guidance and encouragement to meet and be with your baby, you may feel disappointment or hold deep regrets. Perhaps you don't regret not seeing your baby or holding her. That's fine, too. Maybe you were given pain medication that caused you to have a foggy memory. Or maybe you were even the one who refused to see the baby. That happens; parents are sometimes afraid of what the baby will look like or don't know how they will handle a baby who has died. Both meeting and saying goodbye simultaneously are so emotionally draining that perhaps you did not have the energy to do this. No matter the reason, if you hold regrets about refusing pictures and mementos, you can call the labor and delivery department to see if they took any pictures or footprints or handprints. You could meet with one of the nurses or social workers who cared for you. She might be able to fill in the blanks and tell you more about what happened, how your baby looked, who was there, special moments, and so on. Either you or they could write or record these memories so that you will have them as future reminders. Unfortunately, you can't go back, but perhaps you, the staff, and your family can re-create some of your baby's story.

> I know what it is like to live with regrets. We barely saw our son and took no pictures, received no mementos of any kind, and did not invite our family to meet our son. We were in such shock; we made terrible mistakes. I have learned to live with this and had to come to the realization that I did the best I could at the time, and I can't go back. —Sherokee

> Seeing our baby was not an option for so many reasons. We have moved on and don't regret it. It is what it is. —Anonymous

YOU DID YOUR BEST

Surely, you did the best you could in the short time you had. If you made mistakes—most of us do—and have regrets, know that you are not alone. Hopefully, you have some good memories if you saw and held your baby and if your family was included in some way. Again, wanting to rewind the clock and do things differently is extremely common. You may not have received a thorough explanation or you may not have understood information that could have influenced and informed you. But perhaps you had a special, amazing time from the caring, informed staff and other support people, including sacred time spent with your baby. What you have to hold on to is what you have. Cherish it and build from it as you go forward. You can't change the past. Have we said that a few times already?

> We did not know any better, but we sure made some mistakes and hold many regrets even three decades later. We wonder why we didn't invite Brennan's grandparents to the hospital to meet him before we had him cremated. Our siblings wanted to help and be a part of it, too, and we didn't include them in anything where he was present. They never saw him, and even if we had pictures—which we

don't—it is not the same as being there and holding him themselves. —Sherokee

Danielle shared, "I am willing to commit to a lifetime of suffering and pain in hopes that my child has none of that." What a burden for her, as she felt herself lifting the affliction from her child. You may have such feelings, and yet you can't find others who can speak from personal experience about it right now. Hopefully, the stories and vignettes throughout this book will affirm that you are not alone. There are people and resources waiting for you. Heartbreaking Choice is one such Facebook group. More can be found in the resources at the end of this book.

FORGIVENESS AND GRACE

Given everything that has happened, you have come this far and survived. You can only go forward now. So when you can, give yourself grace and forgiveness. Speak with God or your higher power if you have faith and pray through it. Send your child love messages from your heart with your voice, your heart, or in writing. Don't beat yourself up. There was no crystal ball telling you what your child's life would be like, how short it might be, how much pain he would have, or how you as a family would survive. You did the best you could with what you had.

> I have always shared exactly what happened with the loss of my son. People respond with sadness, and I sometimes wonder if they look down on me for the way his life was cut short. But then I realize that it's my own guilt that still seems to seep from my mama heart. I'm learning how to forgive how the death occurred. For me, it was putting my complete trust in God—over and over again. —Jennifer

TIPS AND ADVICE

- Find ways to lighten your burden. Write down any feelings of guilt, shame, blame, and regret. Then tear up the paper, burn it, or bury it.

- Find any decision-making lists you previously created, or make one now. Note the positives of this decision you made for baby and your family. Read it when you have doubts.
- Talk with your partner or someone close to you about your beliefs about abortion and ending a pregnancy. Examine how and why they have changed or not. Get those thoughts and feelings out of your body; don't hold them in.
- Write about any doubts you had—or how you came to a place where there were no doubts—and why. Then put them away for a while (in a box, a drawer, or a deeper corner of your mind). Right now you have much to do to get through this trauma, so put those doubts on hold if you can. You can always come back to them later, if needed.
- Keep a list or a journal of who and what you are grateful for in your life right now. Sometimes you just need to be reminded that all is not dark and difficult. You probably have many blessings in your life. Look at it on those dark days when you feel like there is no tomorrow.
- Say a prayer or seek help from your faith community to help you find peace or use meditation or other means to seek that peace.
- Forgive yourself, and ask for forgiveness. Do not let this decision eat away at you. You have been through so much already.

14

FAMILY DYNAMICS

INTERACTING WITH OTHERS

Following the procedure or induction, meeting your baby (if you were able to do that), and the subsequent good-byes, you may find interacting with others to be a challenge. Your energy may be zapped. Maybe you are still struggling with telling a few people or having unsatisfactory conversations with people who know. You may wonder if you should share what *really* happened or be silent about it. There may be some folks who are rocks for you as you struggle with the days of deep sadness and sorrow. Are you ready to spend time in the outside world, to answer calls, to attend social functions, and even to go back to work? These questions deserve serious consideration as you slowly regain the courage and strength to go forward during dark days.

RESPONSES AND CONVERSATIONS WITH OTHERS

When people respond to you negatively or offer up unhelpful or hurtful advice, give consideration to their previous behaviors and how they handle tough situations and crises. If they tend to give bad advice or seem disrespectful, you may not want to discuss it with them. If, on the other hand, they are usually kindhearted, supportive, and compassionate, you might be willing to have conversations about your loss and the depth of your feelings.

Some parents in this situation choose to limit what they say to strangers and find special ways of talking about it with family and friends. In cases of abortion or pregnancy termination, some parents choose to say their baby was miscarried or stillborn due to genetic problems or maternal issues. They suggest that it keeps things simpler. Or they say that their baby died and that they do not wish to share the details. Or they might feel fine about giving the whole truth since they don't feel embarrassed or guilty about it. You'll need to think about the language you wish to use and the long-term implications, especially if some people know the entire situation and others do not. Secrets usually don't stay quiet.

Your decision may be misunderstood by many people around you. They are on the outside, and no matter how they try to understand what you are going through, they can't. They don't have the same feelings, fears, and pain that you do, yet they want to help and may feel compelled to weigh in on how you should or could go forward. They may be upset and hurting themselves, making it difficult to even approach you, and they may say things without thinking that might cause you pain.

Many other parents in similar situations have been down this road. You can learn from them through websites, books, and even their stories and quotes throughout this book. There are a number of considerations you can take into account as you decide how to interact with others. You will need courage, conviction, support, and reminders of your love as you move forward within your community.

COUPLE COMMUNICATION

What heartbreaking news and stress you have had to endure as a couple! This is not how you envisioned your pregnancy and your family. On the way to a healthy baby and a beautiful future, your life has taken a terrible turn. You had plans for this new life, and instead of a hopeful beginning, there is an unexpected end.

Talking about Guilt and Blame Together

Guilt, blame, and shame often arise, changing the game for couples. Regrets can also creep in. It is likely that one or both of you have had some of these reactions, which can alter your feelings about yourself or one another. Talk this through, read chapter 13, "Regrets and Guilt" together, and give one another grace. It may be that you both have some of the same feelings without realizing it. Maybe you each could make lists about what you feel guilty about. Then over a glass of wine or with some favorite music playing, see how many are found on both lists. If you can get into a playful mood, you could even play charades to get the other person to guess the "guilt" or "blame" scenarios on your list. Some laughter, or at least playfulness, can ease the stress that you are under. Perhaps you could take a walk together (being in nature is healing) and choose not to talk about these feelings. Or you could pick plants and animals that most connect with your feelings. For instance, you might choose a fox because you feel like you have to be sly and secretive around others or a grapevine because you feel like your emotions are so intertwined that you can't sort one feeling from the rest.

No matter what feelings you have, remember that you did the best you could. You are not a bad mother or father for choosing this life-ending path. It was from love and conviction that you are willing to suffer so that you child didn't have to. If this is not affecting you, let it go, move on, and be grateful.

Blaming one another or feeling deep shame impacts your feelings of self and can cause tension and marital stress. Sometimes you may feel that your partner is blaming you by the looks or words that are said, yet your partner may insist that this is not the case. You could be projecting your sense of self-blame onto your partner. Be careful not to do this. It can cause disagreements and fights. Instead, take your partner's word and don't push him or her into a corner where defending actions and feelings becomes a reaction. However, do know that these types of conversations are quite common. How you work through them is key. Through it all, remember that you love one another and that added tension and stress is harmful to both of you and your relationship.

There is much more to read about how men and women grieve and cope in chapter 18, along with a few books written specifically for couples.

SINGLES

As a single mother, you will have your own unique response to this diagnosis and loss. You might be very frustrated that despite modern medicine, your baby could not be cured and you felt compelled to end the pregnancy. With no committed partner and perhaps no other children, you may be upset about being alone again. Even if your support system is good, you may still be overwhelmed with feelings of loss and vulnerability. That is what happens when someone you love dies. It isn't easy to heal and feel healthy again, though it can be done. Naturally, you miss your child and all that you had planned. Unfortunately, you will find that there are many who don't see it quite that way.

Connecting with others who have terminated their pregnancies may be very helpful. You may find it therapeutic to talk with others—including other couples—who have walked in your shoes, even to some degree. You may have trouble with the baby's father and with others who think you should be glad that you are no longer pregnant. Your need for support is great, whether you realize it or not. For more information on these topics, read chapter 19, "Single Moms."

15

HOLDING ONTO MEMORIES

Memories can bring such healing over time for most people. Holding on to the memories of how you told others that you were pregnant and of the gifts and items that were purchased during the pregnancy is a good place to start. You may have written in a diary or journal about the pregnancy, meeting your baby (if you did that), and shared family times after the birth. Hopefully, you collected some mementos and said goodbye in a special way. These are some ways bereaved parents stay connected with their baby over the years. You can do something special on the anniversary of your baby's birth or another significant day to invite others to honor and remember your baby. It could be a picnic at your child's grave or a special park, a cake to celebrate, or donating time at a local charity in memory of your baby. There are many ways to continue to collect memories and mementos.

MEMORIES

Depending upon how you "birthed" your baby—via dilation and curettage (D&C), dilation and evacuation (D&E), or labor and delivery—your mementos, memories, and meeting moment may not be as full as you might wish. However, capture each one and hold it tightly. You cannot live in the past and redo the events, but you can relive it in your mind. You can imagine it as you wish it had been, then repeat that story, write it down, dream it, and make it your own if you wish.

No matter what, you are a mother or father and you do have memories of the pregnancy and the birth experience. Hopefully, you were given time with your baby, offered pictures if possible, and you have some memorable mementos. Even if you feel you did not get enough time seeing and holding your baby, keep in mind that virtually everyone who has a baby who dies says the same thing. There never will be enough time. So as you go back and review that time, you may need to grieve what you feel is lost. When ready, you may also feel gratefulness for that precious time. No one can or should tell you how you should feel at any time; that will be up to you.

> I cherish the clay footprints that the nurses made for me. I also used his ink footprints replicated into a tattoo on my back. —Jennifer

> Even though we did not see a whole baby, I held her within me for those months and buried her remains in a special place. For this I am grateful. —A mom

> I delivered our son at about 22.5 weeks. My husband's parents and my parents were there after he was cleaned up. We baptized the baby, and our parents left after saying their good-byes. We said good-bye about eight hours later and took home a memory box. Looking back, I'm glad we took pictures and had memories, but sometimes I wish we had not included our parents. It was so private, and our son looked so small and dark with death, I almost wish they never had to experience that. —Suzanne

You may be ready to dig into the memory box or read all the cards now. However, if not, do not throw anything away, no matter how upset you might get. Rather, keep an open mind that in the near or far future you will probably want to spend time reviewing your pregnancy, birth, and memories of your baby. This sage advice comes from other parents who have been there and learned the hard way. You may decide later to dispose of some items, but you can do that with wisdom later on, rather than with grief and sadness now.

> I would sit with the memory box for hours in the early weeks touching the small blanket and reading the cards that were sent. I needed to find ways to stay close to her. Though I didn't get to deliver her

whole body, I did get to hold her remains. That meant the world to me. She was my baby and she will be loved forever. —A mom

What follows are a few thoughts about memories and mementos that you might have or could create for your beloved baby, whether she was birthed in labor and delivery or via a D&E.

TIPS AND ADVICE

- Collect all gifts, mementos, clothing, and other items you had for your baby. Handprints and footprints are especially cherished baby items. Put them in a chest, a memory box, or another special place.
- Create a baby album or make a special box or bag with as many mementos as you have. Over time, you can collect more. Save everything, even if you're unsure as to whether you will want it later.
- Memory boxes can be handmade or purchased—a treasure chest, a decorated box from a hobby store, or a wooden or ceramic box. If you or someone close to you is creative, make or find a special box to hold keepsakes.
- Add to the memory box over time. You can store anything from a special outfit, to the names of the first visitors you receive, special books, cards you receive, and so much more. The contents will become tangible memories of your baby's life. You will be able to remember all that she brought into your life, and you will be able to show others, including subsequent children, when the time is right.
- If you sent announcements, wrote in a journal, or have other written mementos, keep them in a special place.
- Collect all pregnancy and sonogram pictures, as well as any photos of the baby. For some people, looking at photos is too difficult at the beginning. If so, tuck them away for now or ask someone you trust to hold them until you are ready.
- Some parents make duplicates of their favorite photos and share them with family members. One reason commonly given is that they worry that if there is ever a fire, these photos are irreplaceable.
- There are many mementos you can buy online or make yourself— bracelets, necklaces, Christmas or holiday ornaments, baby clothes/ blankets, and teddy bears or other stuffed animals. Some people

make bears from a loved one's clothing. If you have a blanket or clothes for your baby already, maybe you could sew a teddy bear or ask someone to do it for you. Grandmother's handkerchiefs or linens could be sewn into a Christmas tree ornament or baby item.

- Plant a tree or flowers that come up every year in memory of your baby. However, be mindful that they can't be taken with you. For example, if planting a tree, consider whether you might move in the future.
- Some parents send bulbs or flowers to family members to plant in hopes that when they grow the following year, the baby will be on their minds.
- Donate baby toys to a local charity. Ask your family to do the same.
- Spend time on the Internet looking at personalized mementos such as lockets, jewelry, charms, necklaces, and bears/dolls.
- Create some sort of legacy that lives on to honor your baby. It could be a fundraising walk, an annual donation to the hospital or a baby loss charity, a book drive for favorite books to be donated to the hospital or clinic, a fund to help pay for funerals for other families, and so on. There is so much that can be done to help others and to remember your little one. And there are many needy baby loss charities that you can support, so carefully consider whether you need to start one. You may be able to work with an existing one and include your baby's name.
- Remember, too, that you can always name the baby and have a service inviting family members to say good-bye and gather together at a later date. A service can be just as special and personal whether your baby's body is present or not.
- If you did not get to deliver your baby but had a procedure that didn't provide a whole baby to hold and take pictures of, you may feel that there are few memories to cherish and very little to put in a memory box. You may be able to retrieve ultrasound pictures or videos, notes from your chart, mementos given at the hospital or that were purchased later, pregnancy photos, pregnancy casts, and more. You can also continue to add to the box over time. Although this is yet another loss, it doesn't mean that you need to forget your baby and the time you were pregnant with her. You'll just have to try a little harder. Think about the pregnancy memorabilia that you could

put together, such as pregnancy photos, pregnancy casts, and three-dimensional ultrasound videos.

- In time, you may look at life differently and realize how important relationships are, given life's fragility. Maybe your baby's life touched someone deeply, and they are changed in profound ways. Many families become altruistic, creating a legacy that lives on. Parents may start or participate in a run or walk that honors their baby. Some join organizations, start websites, donate baby items, or provide self-help materials to other families in need. Others may move on privately without taking on any new projects, living with the memories they have and hold in their hearts. Your baby's short life can become a springboard for any number of gifts as you seek your new normal, see beauty and love in the world in a new way, and change your attitude and behaviors in amazing ways. These are gifts that come from and because of your baby.

III

Continuing Your Healing Journey

As time goes by, you will find many considerations arise for you and your family. In the early days you will be in the middle of the devastation. Couple and family dynamics can be influenced by one another's beliefs and experiences. Your personalities and how you were raised impact how you interact and go forward. If you have other children, their ongoing needs and behaviors may challenge you to try different ideas and to learn more about how children develop. Workplace issues, starting with decisions about whether you or your partner go back to work or how you go back to work, are important considerations.

Some discussion and reading about typical grief reactions may help you to better work toward healing. Being a "good" griever and trusting your instincts are two good places to start. Chapter 23, "Grief and Healing" has many thoughts and suggestions; you'll also find many books in the resources at the end of this book.

As you integrate your grief into your life, you'll see healing and painful reminders in your journey toward healing. We affirm what is well known: that you will never forget and that you will always love your baby but that grief will come and go, hopefully lessening over time as you work at it.

Having another baby may or may not be something you want to do. Chapter 25, "Trying Again," is written for those who do want to try again. But of course there are no guarantees that having another baby is in your future. We are careful to point out that having another baby is not the magical answer for healing. The process of loving and remembering the babies who died still continues even when your arms are filled with another child. This is a reality of life. There are no easy and permanent solutions for mending a broken heart. However, there are ways to go forward that soften the pain and add beauty and love back into your life.

16

THE EARLY DAYS

After having a baby die or a child born with multiple challenges, your view of the world has changed. Previously, you may have reveled in the joy of meeting other pregnant women. Your friends may have spent hours talking about pregnancy, birth, and babies with you. The world revolves around the pregnancy when one is living it. Thus, it makes sense that there is pain and confusion when interacting with friends, relatives, and acquaintances after your baby has died.

PREGNANT WOMEN

Seeing or being with pregnant women can be very hard in the early days. You may not know how to deal with the news or the sight of others' pregnancies. This can be especially true if they were pregnant at the same time or on the same cycle as you. Whether it is a friend, relative, neighbor, work colleague, or even a stranger, you may get upset or want to check out. Sometimes a physical response even overtakes you. Your emotions may fire up and surprise you. Some mothers talk of the excruciating pain that keeps them from shopping. Picking up your children from school or returning to work may also be difficult. Reminders of what you no longer have, but others do, is like salt in your wound. This is a new perspective you never planned for, but it is your new reality.

As a father, this may not affect you as it does your partner. You may hurt for her when she tells you how her heart aches when she sees a baby or a mother-to-be. It is almost an unconscious, instinctual response. If you don't feel this, you probably can't understand. But trust that it is real for her. You may have your own reactions; sometimes anger that not having your baby with you hurts you both so much. Some fathers have explained that they felt helpless when it came to supporting their partners. You may feel this if you are one who seeks to fix things and to solve problems. It seems so easy and perfect for others, but not for you. It is true; there are so many ways that you have been cheated of the many plans you had for the future. You don't get to throw your baby in the air, teach him how to throw and catch a ball, and use that toy box that you built. You will miss the first day of kindergarten, fishing trips together after hunting for worms, and camping trips and sporting events that would have created special memories for both of you. This may feel like salt in *your* wound, yet you may put it away for now or for a long time. Many dads feel their first priority is to take care of their partners. Mothers don't understand this, just as you may not understand her empty, aching arms and tears about not having had the opportunity to breastfeed.

> It's been just over a year now and I feel different. More tired and even a bit tearful. Sadness is combined with anger and I can't get a grip. What I realize is that I have held it all in while I took care of my wife. Now that she is getting better and laughs out loud again, it seems that it is my turn. Now I feel the grief coming on. But whom will I talk with about it? Others expected me to be over it the first few weeks. —A dad

Both of you will feel cheated and maybe even bitter. Your plans were interrupted and this setback can't be fixed. That's frustrating for men who need jobs to do in a crisis and who genuinely want to know what can be done to help their partners. If you go to a support group or like to be online, you may find help from other fathers. Your clergy or a counselor might have insight and there are books written by men that might help you deal with your own feelings and find your style of coping.

EMPTY ARMS

While others continue to enjoy their babies after yours died or suffers serious problems, your arms are empty. If your baby still lives, your basket may be full of complications and problems. Envy, jealousy, and sadness—no matter how bad they may sound—are normal emotions in this situation. You may need to think about how to handle this. Will you shop online for a while rather than go to the mall? Should you take a different route so that you don't drive right past the daycare your child would have attended? You may avoid baby showers and baptisms for a while. For a time, you can use these strategies to minimize the pain in your heart, but eventually you will find ways to deal with and soften the pain. Maybe you'll talk with others or write your feelings down in order to get those feelings out. You might need to spend time with a pregnant friend; if you feel safe, you can share your feelings and work to get over this obstacle so the next time is not as difficult.

> Shortly after Brennan was born, I needed to hold a baby. Although I knew it would be the next hardest thing in the world (after living through his death, that is), I needed my arms filled with a baby, and I wanted to be able to face moms and babies. I went to my friend's house and spent about a half hour there. She allowed me to hold her baby who was born within days of Brennan. I cried, she cried, and we talked a bit. In retrospect, it must have been hard for her, too. It could have been her baby. What if the roles were reversed? I must say, it took much courage to do this, but I was so glad I did. I felt cleansed and a bit renewed to face a new day and another newborn.
> —Sherokee

DAILY LIFE

Believe it or not, one of the most feared places for many parents in your situation is the grocery store. From the clerk to the people you know, from the baby aisle to the impatience of standing in line—you may need to put on your armor and dig deep for your courage the first few times you go back. People may ask about your pregnancy or baby and you may see other babies. Simply seeing baby products can break your heart. Some mothers choose to avoid stores in the early days of their loss.

When others asked how they could help, the moms made lists and the friend or relative did the shopping. This is not a long-term answer, but it might help during some of the difficult times.

When people call your home, you have some choices. You could ask good friends or family to be there to answer for you. Another option is to record a message such as, "Thank you for calling and caring. We have had a significant loss and are doing everything we can to take care of ourselves. If you leave us a message, we may or may not call you back. Please be understanding if we just can't get to it." Or you could say, "We are either not home or are busy right now. Given the circumstances, don't expect a call back from us."

When you do feel ready to answer a call, you can, but your bases are covered when or if you can't. You could also have a note posted on your front door when you are home alone and just can't answer. It could say something like, "If you are leaving something for us, feel free to put it in the basket. We are either gone or busy right now and choosing not to answer our door. Thanks for understanding."

Friends and family want to help. Let them. There may be other things they can do, such as organize dinner, take care of the other children, clean the house, and take care of you.

When you are back at work, you will have to face coworkers and maybe even the public. This can be a challenge. If you can contact your supervisor prior to returning and make some arrangements, you may find it easier to return. Hopefully, you will receive support. If not, you'll have some decisions to make. Some of your considerations might be whether you continue working there, change your attitude, or attempt to obtain a leave of absence.

> I found it really hard to go back to work even a month after our loss. I worked for a call center where I was expected to be patient and polite with customers. I couldn't imagine going back, knowing I could care less about someone's Internet problems. But we needed the money and I had to go back. My supervisor gave me a little wiggle room for breaks and [allowed me] to pass hard calls on. In the end, I realized I had to suck it up and just do my work. In some ways, it kept my mind busy, so [it] wasn't so bad. In other ways, it was hard, but not as hard as burying my daughter. This is life, I guess. It goes on, no matter what. —A mom

17

BUILDING SUPPORT FROM OTHERS

As the days and weeks go by, it may seem hard to adapt to your new life with no baby or with a baby who has significant needs. Your energy may be focused on your nuclear family now, but there are so many other things to do, from mundane tasks like shopping and paying bills to driving other children to activities and planning for upcoming holidays. You may think you must do these things alone, but many people are waiting anxiously in the wings, ready and waiting to be asked for help.

RECEIVING SUPPORT

You may have parents, siblings, good friends, and others who "get it" and who are doing everything they can to support you and to show love for and to honor your baby, no matter the news. Cherish these people and keep them included during the months ahead. Keep the dialogue open and ask them to check in with you when they have suggestions or concerns. You can do this in person, via phone or text, or even e-mail or social media. When you share this part of the journey with them, chances are good that they will be there for you—and each other—in the challenging days ahead.

Never assume that people have lost interest or don't care because they don't check in frequently or because you haven't heard from them in awhile. Perhaps, out of respect, they don't want to trouble you, so they wait for cues from you. Perhaps they are trying to help you to focus and talk about other things to keep your mind occupied or to limit what they see as "negative thoughts." They might invite you to the movies, gatherings, or talk of ordinary things.

You may misunderstand or be confused by some people's responses to you when you tell them about your path. They may not understand your choice and may appear judgmental, no matter which direction you took. They view it from the outside and are not living it like you. Even though they hurt and may be deeply concerned, they don't have the same feelings, fears, and pain that you do; yet they want to help and may feel compelled to offer guidance about moving forward. The words and advice they offer may not help. If you can, accept that they are trying, but understand that they can't read your mind and don't really know how to help, so they are making it up as they go based on what they think you might like or what they think they would want others to do for them.

There may be some people who tried to discourage you from continuing or from ending your pregnancy, and you may be concerned about what they think about you now. Keep in mind that their opinions usually are voiced out of love and a sense of protection; they do not want you to suffer, but they don't know how to prevent that. They feel at a loss about how to help you. Many parents have felt judged by others, by those who said they understood why they had no choice but to make the decision they made. Parents are the hardest on themselves. Try to lighten up on yourself and on others if you can. Don't allow tension and misunderstandings among family and friends create more losses and pain.

Think of people you know who are naturally positive and supportive. Then surround yourself with them. If you are not sure who they are, review their previous behaviors. How others handle delicate subjects and crises will help provide insight about who those people are.

In the likely event that you feel the need to talk, try to choose someone who you know will care and who has previously shown themselves to be a good listener. The following suggestions are to help you assist others in understanding and respecting your unique situation and choices. You may wonder, "Why should I help others to process and accept my child's diagnosis? Shouldn't they be helping me instead?" Given that they probably don't know how to help, this is your chance to share something that will enlighten them. Maybe these ideas will positively impact their attitudes about your pregnancy and your precious baby.

Remember that at the end of the day, you have to live with your choices while others will move on with their lives. Just as you were shocked by the news, so your family and friends may be. Give them time and help them to come to terms with the situation.

TIPS AND ADVICE FOR FRIENDS

- The following tips are for the friends and family of someone who has experienced a loss.
- Be supportive. Be present. Share ideas or ways to help rather than asking what you can do to help. Parents who have had a loss may not have a clue about what they need.
- Speak the baby's name out loud if the baby was named. If you are not sure what the family wants, ask if they named the baby and if it is okay to refer to him by name.
- Mom and dad are parents and they always will be. Treat them as such. Their child may not be here on Earth, but he is present in their hearts forever. The baby was always loved, and he happened to have died, but he continues to be loved.
- Be thoughtful, sensitive, compassionate, and loving. Please don't add to their burden of pain. If you can't do that immediately, write them a kind note that expresses your concern and stay away if you think you'll be tempted to say something that won't be helpful.
- Listen to mom and dad. Invite them to talk about their experience. Hold their hands. Cook them a meal.
- Don't avoid them or the subject unless the parents specifically ask you to not talk about it.
- Learn more about their situation so that you are better prepared to help. You can contact organizations that help with child loss and ask for helpful bereavement information and materials.
- Visit the library or spend time looking at credible Internet sources. When you know more, it may become more obvious how to offer support and help. Just be careful not to overwhelm them with what you've learned. If you have something to share, you could offer an overview and ask if they want to know the source or ask you more. If

they prefer to take in small bits of information, respect that. They are coping the best way they know how.

- Don't judge them, no matter their decisions. You never know how you would handle such an awful situation unless you are there yourself. No one can prepare you for this, and there is no easy solution.
- Treat them respectfully, as friends, rather than as freaks or bad people who made a bad choice.
- Within the next few months and years, your friends or family will grieve their baby's death, but there will also be days when they are feeling better and would love to do something or to talk about something else. Invite them to join you in a normal activity sometime, but don't press them if they are not able or interested at that time. When they are ready, they will join you.
- If you have advice to offer, ask if they would like to hear it. If not, hold it back for now.
- Don't give them the impression they should "get over" their feelings.
- Don't dwell on how their child died or the decision they had to make. The fact remains that they are here now and need compassion and love.
- Remember their other children and help however you are able.
- Know that words will not ease the pain, though they can add to the pain if they are insensitive.
- Avoid using a higher being's "will" to justify or explain the death. That is for them to decide, not you.
- Be patient, even if they seem withdrawn or angry at times.
- Be sensitive to the fact that they may not want to see or hold babies in the same age group as their child.
- The support of friends and family plays a vital part in this journey. Such love and support makes a huge difference in parents' lives. There are many other sources of support, such as support groups for parents going through the same experience.
- If you find such resources, share them. Be courageous and step up to the plate. If you don't, who will? What if it were you? What would you want to happen?

DEALING WITH UNKIND, UNHELPFUL WORDS

There will be people who either directly or indirectly say things that add pain to your heart. They may not even realize it. It might be that they don't know what to say or how to be supportive, so things come out of their mouths without much thought of how they may be received.

Given what has happened, you are definitely vulnerable to the behavior and comments of others. Even if they don't mean to hurt you—and most don't—your heightened sensitivity and fear of being judged may cause you to take thoughtless comments more seriously than you otherwise would. Comments by others can add to your own guilt and sadness. You are grieving and sensitive.

> I cannot forget the comment an acquaintance made to me at the funeral of my daughter. She was silently crying so I went to see if she was okay. She proceeded to tell me that her dog had gotten run over that morning and so she understood: "we were both burying our babies today." It took superhuman strength not to go hysterical on her! —Stephanie

> About four months after our interruption, a friend who had gone through two unsuccessful in vitro fertilization treatments and finally adopted asked if I was going to attend an event celebrating the Indian New Year. I explained that I did not feel ready, especially because in our community I would get more questions about what happened. She told me, "You need to get thicker skin and let it roll off." I don't remember my response, but I know that I have not talked to her since. —B.T.

TIPS AND ADVICE FOR YOU

- Refer to your child by his or her name if you selected a name. This makes him or her real, human, and a member of the family and highlights the fact that you are having a real, loved son or daughter, no matter what happens or when.
- Do what you can to show that this is your baby, not an event to "get over." You will always be the parent of this child, even though he or

she may die or have challenges. The more you can show life, love, and legacy, the more likely others will begin to understand you.

- Write a letter or send an e-mail to others (you could write one and make copies) telling them what is happening and ways that you hope they can be helpful.

- Ask your clergy, church family, neighbors, and extended family to reach out to the people around you who may need guidance as to how to respond to the situation. They may give them advice about how to behave and what they can do to help, especially if you feel overwhelmed and don't have the energy to do it.

- Work to understand and forgive those who just can't, or won't, be there for you. It is hard to know why some people retreat and are silent. Maybe they are at a loss for words, have little energy to give right now, or carry emotional baggage or issues that make it painful to be there for you now, even if they want to. There are plenty of reasons why people don't step up and help. You'll have to decide if you can let it go and forgive, either now or in the future.

- Work toward understanding and forgiveness.

- Try to see things in a positive light. Assume the best about others; at least they are trying. After all, they could ignore you and not even try to reach out to you. Chances are, you already have had experience with this with others.

- Document unhelpful and hurtful comments and how you feel about them, which may feel good, then you tear them up afterward.

- Respond with kindness, even if it is hard. For example, you could say, "I am sorry, but I need to tell you that that does not help me. I wish you might have said something more positive and affirming like 'This must be so hard. I am here for you.'" Or "I trust you don't mean to, but that comment hurts me. When I hear that, I have doubts and even some shame about what we did. Hopefully, you don't want to add more pain to my hurting heart." Or "I know you can't know what I have been through; therefore, I will give grace and forgiveness by not taking what you have said to heart."

- Remember that at the end of the day, you have to live with yourself and with your choices while others will move on with their lives. Just as you were shocked by the news, so your family and friends may be. Give them time and help in coming to terms with the situation if you are able, and seek support from those who understand, especially parents who have been there. They may become your greatest support system. You can find them in the resources provided at the end of this book. You may also ask your genetic counselor, social worker, hospital caregivers, clergy, or others to help you network with parents in your community who have made similar heartbreaking choices.

18

HOW MEN AND WOMEN GRIEVE AND GET ALONG

Reaching agreement on important, life-altering decisions is never easy—for anyone. Some couples find agreement quickly; many do not. Whether you and your partner were in sync or you spent hours in discussion with tension and disagreement, the bottom line is that you love your baby and that this is your new path. There is no turning back, whether you were in full agreement or not. The next phase is keeping your relationship strong while navigating the aftermath of your decision.

RELATIONSHIPS TAKE WORK

You may feel your relationship has been put to the test. This roller coaster has taken a toll on your relationship; you will need to work together to stay strong. Relationships take work, especially when under stress. On the other hand, if you were on the same page regarding your tough decision, you may feel that at least you move side by side into tomorrow. During this time, you may find patience short, anger common, and deep sadness abundant. All of these emotions bring challenges for the calm, peace, and acceptance you may seek. Such internal struggles can result in external outbursts and couple confusion. Don't let them ruin a beautiful family. And even if you have issues—and who doesn't?—you can choose to work through them. Or maybe you are

fine, mostly on the same page, and offering one another comfort and
support.

UNDERSTANDING ONE ANOTHER

Seeking to understand one another better might help you as you move
ahead. Men and women differ in many respects, particularly when it
comes to emotional issues. As you faced the fact that your child had a
poor or fatal condition, you were influenced by your past attitudes and
behaviors to various life stresses before the diagnosis. Chances are you
will still do so afterward. Whether it is your unique personality style,
upbringing, fears, or frustrations, you will see the world through your
own glasses, not your partner's. Therefore you may not quite understand what your partner is thinking or wants.

> The biggest thing a man can do is to listen to his wife/partner. You
> need to have your ears open and hold your partner. Listen and don't
> judge them. Let them grieve. It was good to read the Bible, but I dug
> my head into it and overdid it. Women accept things and men have
> to fix things. I did the best I knew how to do at the time—asking God
> to fix it because He is a healing God. But while He gives, He also
> takes away. I tried to go to God and fix things. But while I was
> soaking all that scripture in, I neglected Angie and Cyrus in a way. In
> a lot of ways, I caused more hurt than healing at that time because I
> was so bent on Titus being healed that I forgot to love throughout
> that time. Faith is good, but faith is not the greatest thing. Love is.
> —Cecil, *Giant Hero*

Although many will say there are no right or wrong ways to react and
behave, there are in fact better ways and less helpful ways. Some ways
are hurtful or harmful to relationships. For example, if one of you wants
to talk and the other refuses, this can cause trouble unless each of you
understands what is really going on. If one of you is highly emotional
much of the time and the other is calm and reserved, you may make
judgments about whether your partner is coping in a healthy manner
(because she or he is not coping like you are). It is detrimental to your
relationship if one of you is angry and hurting yourself or your partner.
Do everything you can to keep the communication channels open. Ima-

gine you are in your partner's shoes. What would you feel or do if you were him or her? When you are unsure, ask.

COUPLE RELATIONSHIPS

Ordinary conversation and outright happiness may seem long gone. For some couples, nothing seems ordinary now. Some couples find their loss brings them closer together as they comfort and work to understand one another. And if you are sensitive and kindhearted, at least you aren't adding to the pain. Nurture and care for one another knowing that you are both hurting and missing your child or grieving the loss of a healthy child. The more you can learn about how men and women grieve, the better.

> Our relationship went through many trials after the loss. I shut down and turned to creating an online memorial for my daughter. A couple of months after the loss, our relationship hit a breaking point. We realized that we needed each other more than ever to lean on, and our relationship was better than ever. —Emma

> I feel that the relationship between my husband, Mark, and I has become even stronger. We have seen one another in our depths of despair and been so proud of one another for how we handled everything. We have always had so much love for one another but now it's extra special when we can see some of Gabrielle when we look at one another. However, there were times after Gabrielle passed away when we were a little tense with one another. Being stressed and emotional can blow little things out of proportion. —Gabrielle's mom

GOING OUT IN PUBLIC

Going out in public may be very painful and awkward for one or both of you. How do each of you answer the inevitable questions about your pregnancy? "Weren't you pregnant?" "Where is your baby?" "Oh, how sad. What happened?" "How is your wife doing?" A natural response is to simply stay home for a while—why not avoid the public for a while?

This makes some sense. You need to let the grief flow and you may not be ready to be out there in public yet; privacy has some advantages. However, hiding out in your safety zone can't last forever; there will be reasons for you to go out. Some preparation and a willingness to dig deep for the courage can help you. This can become especially complicated if one of you seems ready or willing to go out to gatherings but the other does not. It is important to communicate with one another about your needs, desires, and the reasons for them. You will want to compromise sometimes and give in to the other at least a little. If you each start going in different directions and holding hard feelings about it, you can be sure your relationship is not headed in the right direction. To help you with this you could seek counseling, have "dinner talk nights," send one another e-mails or texts, or write one another love notes. Give your partner the benefit of the doubt when interpreting his or her messages, even if it doesn't come across as positive as you might wish.

One or both of you may need to get back to work soon due to company policies, your need to *do* something, financial pressures, or other reasons. If one partner is home, it is easy for him or her to feel abandoned and alone. What do you do all day if you don't have other children there? And what do you do if you have other children around but don't have the energy or patience to care for them? Don't just plunge back into the work scene before talking about it. Make some plans and create a transition plan if possible. Maybe working part time or coming home for lunch would be most beneficial. Perhaps inviting a relative or friend to help with the children or to keep your partner company might help. Ask others for ideas. It is important to find something that works for both of you.

FATHER AND MOTHERS GRIEVE DIFFERENTLY

Your family and community's beliefs may fall into the stereotype that views mother as shattered on the floor and father as the steadying force who lifts and carries her during this difficult time. Many men in many cultures have been taught that men don't cry, that they don't love their unborn children as much as mother does, that their wives will crumble if they see their husbands cry, and that strength and courage need to be shown but can't be combined with tears, which show weakness. These messages can make it hard for men to express their feelings to others or even to themselves. They can also be the seeds that create disharmony because women may interpret this apparent lack of emotion as a sign of not loving the baby enough. Resentment and misunderstanding can occur easily between partners unless there is strong communication and an openness to discuss and respect each partner's differences and similarities. Don't make your partner's ways of coping or of feeling emotion wrong or right; they are what they are for each person.

Many women prefer to talk, reviewing what has happened and how they feel. Men often choose to be busy, hoping to move ahead and avoid the pain. It may be they don't know what else to do. Since many mothers want to talk about the baby, as well as their hopes and dreams, it is imperative that you find ways to do this occasionally with your partner and with others. Don't force him to be present every time you need to wallow unless he wants to. What he may really want is to solve the problem for you. Unfortunately this is a problem that cannot be fixed.

Although you both love your baby, you very well may have different needs and strategies for coping with the loss. Common sense and stress impacts relationships, especially when emotions run high. Go forward while making the most of the time you had with your baby. Relive and hold dear all the memories and mementos you have. Focus on what really matters now—your relationship, your mental and physical health, and your other children if you have any. Make an agreement with one another not to spend much—or any—time revisiting the stress of the decision and who said or did what. You can't undo any of that, and you don't need regrets negatively impacting your journey forward. Let them go, if you can. Write them down and tear them up. Spend time in nature and think or pray them away. Lighten your burden. Seek the light whenever you can.

There are a few books and booklets that might be helpful to you, including *Couple Communication after a Baby Dies* by Sherokee Ilse and Tim Nelson, *For Better, For More* by Maribeth Doerr, and *Grieving Parents— Surviving Loss As a Couple* by Nathalie Himmelrich. With practical advice, stories, and humor, these books may help you to learn quite a bit about one another if you read and discuss them as you go. These books are listed in resources at the end of this book.

The following are a few tips to consider as you enter the next leg of this unexpected journey beyond your loss.

TIPS AND ADVICE

- Good communication skills are a mixture of expressing your feelings and needs *and* listening to your partner's.
- Be open to the other's ideas and thoughts. They may not be at all like yours, but you might find that insightful dialogue comes from truly listening to your partner.
- Give one another some undivided attention each day. During that time, minimize distractions like the television, phone, and computer. Plan an hour of "together time" to talk or just to *be*.
- When you say something important, ask your partner to repeat what she or he heard. Then you do the same. Work to reduce the number of misunderstandings.
- Speak from your own heart, saying "I" more than "you," which can sound accusatory or put your partner on the defensive.
- Some people are not good at communicating verbally through words. If this is the case, use other methods such as writing e-mails or texts, leaving phone messages, or even handwriting your thoughts and needs. This can strip some of the emotions from your exchanges.
- If you have a pet, spend time together or alone with him or her. Pets can be therapeutic. They take you out of your own mind and into another space. Walking, petting, and playing with your pet can be calming and helpful.
- Each of you may have your own emotional baggage and past hurts. When stressed, that baggage and those previous feelings can resurface, further complicating your loss. You will notice that your current emotions combine with past ones, sometimes adding to feelings of being overwhelmed.
- One or both of you may still have doubts about the decision you made. If you decide to air what you are thinking, be very careful about insinuating that you hold it against your partner.
- As another way to process things when you disagree, write your partner's concerns (or fears, desires, or needs) in a notebook or on a small whiteboard. You are finished only when your partner agrees

that you properly captured their feelings. Then take turns. This helps with good listening and careful communication and minimizes exaggeration and assumptions.

- Focus on the present and the issues, concerns, or decisions that are needed now or in the near-term. Don't get too far ahead of yourself if you are easily overwhelmed, which is very common. Table less immediate issues until the point at which you have to deal with them.
- Spend some time together going over memories, looking at mementos, and recalling any rituals you had when with your baby. These can change over time as you become more comfortable.
- If you do think that you need some help, ask a relative or friend to do some research for you. For example, you might want help making a memory box or planning an event to honor your child. Maybe you need to find resources and others to talk with.
- Talk with a counselor who has experience with infant death and decision making. Conduct an interview ahead of time to be sure. Not all therapists are trained in this area and they can do more harm than good. However, don't wait until things fall apart so badly they cannot be pieced back together. Think of it as preventative maintenance for your marriage.
- Maintain respect and take breaks when you need them. You can focus on problem solving for only so long. Have some fun if you can allow it. Even a little goes a long way.
- Watch some movies and television shows that make you laugh. Laughter and levity can definitely provide a short release from stress and strain.
- Exercise is vital to staying healthy. If you have any concerns about exercise, check with your doctor before starting any new exercise program. Drink lots of water and eat nutritious food. Help one another to accomplish this every day if you can.
- Don't expect your partner—or anyone—to read your mind. Say what you want out loud or write a note. Don't be upset because you wanted something to happen but your partner didn't come through. This adds more disappointment and trauma to an already difficult situation.
- Develop or create a physical sign like rubbing your thumb on your nose, crossing your eyes, or making a circle with your finger and thumb as a code. Use this physical sign to silently convey when you

want your partner to help you stop a conversation, when children are listening nearby, or when you want to avoid answering the door and dealing with a nosey neighbor.

- Spend some time in nature together. Barefoot. Throw a ball or Frisbee to one another. Sit on the grass cross-legged and tell stories. Make S'mores over a fire. Get out of the house and into different scenery.
- Forgive one another for failings and mistakes.
- Mostly, listen to one another. Remember that you are both suffering and that you love one another.
- Remember to spend time with others, as well, and to give one another a break. If you were ones to go out separately now and then, continue to do so. Continue your other friendships, and give one another space to continue to pursue individual interests.

19

SINGLE MOMS

COMMENTS BY OTHERS

Be prepared for questions about your baby and subsequent comments regarding your loss. You probably know all too well what they are already: "You're young; you'll bounce back"; "It wasn't meant to be"; "Now you can go back to dating [or being a kid, or being *free*] again"; "God spared you a lifetime of pain and sorrow"; "Not having a husband would have made it harder—at least you won't be burdened by a lifetime of expensive care"; "You couldn't really afford a baby right now, anyway; this is better for you"; and "Now you can go to college and get a fresh start." You know the drill. Maybe you have even said some of these things to yourself. The difference is, you are the parent, so you are allowed to say and feel as you wish. Others should not be offering insensitive platitudes as consolation or giving questionable advice to you. However, most people do it out of concern, protection (of you and them), and because they don't know any better or don't know what else to say. Don't let these comments get to you. They know not what they say or the impact it has on you.

TROUBLE WITH THE BABY'S FATHER

If you are having troubles with the father of your baby, you are not alone. Many dads do step up and support mom during this horrible time. However, there are also many who can't deal with it and leave. Or they come and go, making an already difficult time more confusing. It's possible he doesn't have the skills and coping style to be with you during these difficult times. Some men are not good at this in general. They may not have learned how to express deep emotional pain or support others at such times. Or they just may not be comfortable in this realm of life. There may be past experiences that resurface causing anxiety and fear. You really don't know why he can't be there for you now; you just know that's how it is. Although you cannot change your baby's father and the troubles he is having, you can change how you deal with him. If he is causing you additional stress, get help from others to get away from or to distance yourself from him. Ask for some time to take care of yourself and get your health back. Don't respond to angry or hurtful texts or calls. Find a counselor to offer you support and guidance.

> My husband was in Iraq when I got the news. We tried to get him a medical leave but they told him maybe he could come home when the baby was born, not before. I had to endure the rest of my pregnancy without him. It stunk! Thankfully, my mother or sister came with me to every appointment and helped me live through the long five months. We had to take videos and use Skype to communicate, and I even had to have the birth videotaped because he didn't get home. I felt so alone, but we made it. We both have lots of regrets that we are learning to live with. Sometimes you have to make sacrifices and then move on. We try to be positive as much as possible. We'll always be little Sammy's mommy and daddy. —A mom

If you have a same-sex partner, the same issues may apply. One of you is likely more emotional and open about expressing feelings and needs, while the other may hold it in and deal with problems and crises intellectually. Working to communicate when you can about what is important and allowing past problems or petty concerns go for now is helpful.

No matter what has happened or how it happened, you are here now. You have made it so far. You will find ways to cope. Hopefully, you will also find people who offer supportive comments and thoughtful advice when you need it and who are there when you need them. Go forward with hope and a commitment that you will make it, that you are not alone, and that your baby will always be with you.

I wish [my baby's father] hadn't left me. Yeah, it *is* hard, but now he has made it harder for *me*. I have to do it alone. I focus too much on him, wanting him to be here and to give me comfort. But he can't and he won't. He left, so now I have to find others. Social media has been a lifesaver in the middle of the night. Even though some people say really stupid things, most of the time it's been good to know I am not alone. —Isabelle

SEEKING HELP FROM OTHERS

How do you find help? Look within your circle of family and friends and ask yourself who has stood by you before. Find someone who does not judge you harshly or undermine your decisions. Think of what you may specifically need from someone and look for those types of qualities among those in your circle as you consider who to ask for support. Maybe you need a calm presence or someone who will be honest but not brutal with you. A stable character or an assertive communicator might be helpful. Make your list and seek out your support system. Then invite them to be on your "team" during the days and weeks ahead.

You may find—or could create—a Facebook group of other singles who are facing challenges in their pregnancies. You can be sure they are out there, though they may not be as numerous as couples facing those issues. Having friends who are couples during this time helps, especially if they have had similar experiences. Helping you might be very therapeutic and special for them.

There are a few resources out there for you. Connie Nykiel has written *After the Loss of Your Baby: For Teen Mothers* and Sherokee Ilse is the author of *Single Parent Grief*, another booklet that offers advice and support.

With help from my support group leader who was also my nurse, I have come to realize that as a teen mom, I also deserve understanding and love. Sure, I made a mistake getting pregnant in the first place, but I wouldn't go back. I am Jake's mommy and I always will be. Now I want to help other teen moms. I just don't know where to start. —A teen mom

TIPS AND ADVICE

- Surround yourself with positive people who do not judge you for having a baby when you are young or without a partner and who will be sources of positive support.
- Be assertive and let others know what is helpful or not helpful with what they're doing or saying to you.
- Take time out. Single parents find it much harder to have "me time," but it is very important to both your physical and mental health.
- Exercise every day. You can walk, jump on a trampoline (which is good for boosting your immune system), run, do Pilates or Zumba, or visit the gym for a good workout. Exercise increases the endorphins in your system, which can help you to feel better emotionally and physically.
- Meditate or do yoga.
- Pray and ask others to pray for you.
- Spend time with pets, yours or a friend's. Pets are great therapy when you are grieving.
- Buy yourself soft tissues for your tears and candles and inspirational music for your quiet moments.
- Set aside time for your grief or view it as time to be with your baby in spirit. Set a specific time, such as one hour in the evening, then prepare what you need (tissues, candles, music, baby mementos, cards you were sent, paper to write on or tear up, etc.). Set the timer then spend your time thinking and reviewing. When time is up, put your things away, dry your tears, and move on to something else. Compartmentalizing like this may help you to stop feeling sad all the time and to stop feeling guilty when you are not sad. You can make such an appointment each day, knowing that you have scheduled your "baby remembering time." But you should also know that it is okay—and possible—to have some ordinary living time without feeling guilty.
- Surround yourself with a team of people (or even just a few committed friends) who believes in you, wants to help, is trustworthy, and gives good guidance and support.
- Stay positive. Send out positive energy and ask others to send you positive energy.

- Join a support group for single parents. There is a value in talking to those who have "walked the walk" and who genuinely understand what you may be going through.
- Keep a list of things and people for whom you are grateful. Or put notes into a gratitude jar (a container you can decorate to hold your notes). Write down at least one thing for which you are grateful each day. On days when you are feeling low, read some. This may remind you that all is not dark or painful in your life.
- Look for a supportive mental health professional. Not all health professionals are created the same, and it is important to choose one who will be supportive of your age, relationship, situation, or whatever it might be. Connecting with the right therapist for you is so important.
- Finally, be kind to yourself. Being single through this journey can be difficult. But one thing is certain: it does not change how much you love your little one and how beautiful you both are. Be gentle and patient with yourself.

20

SUPPORTING YOUR CHILDREN

If you have other living children, you may have given deep considera-tion about how you present the sad news to them and how you engage them at the time of your loss. You likely also have questions and con-cerns about how to help them over time.

BEING THERE FOR YOUR CHILDREN

The loss of your beloved baby is not only a tragedy for you, but it is also a traumatic and confusing time for your children as well. You are full of shock, sadness, and intense grief. But you wish to be there for your other children. At some point, they need to be included and informed about what has happened to their brother or sister. Even if they are young, they know that something important has happened. Most ex-perts agree that you should not keep them in the dark unless they are very young or they didn't know you were pregnant. As hard as it is to say the words to your children, you will find a way to face them and to be honest. One mother shared that she did not tell her children that the baby died, hoping that when she was pregnant again she could pretend it was the same baby. This kind of thinking can be problematic and may lead to distrust in the days ahead.

How you tend your children and work to meet their needs during this chaotic, painful time is worth thinking about. It may not be easy to give of yourself if you feel spent and exhausted. If your child is acting out—which often happens when there is a change in routine or tension in the home—you will recognize that parenting an upset child is difficult on a good day when you are well. Now you are hurting and not thinking clearly. You may be in bed or unable to care for even basic needs at times. Seek help from family and friends whom you trust with your children. Hopefully they can lighten your burden during the early days of your loss. And do your best to sit with them and even just hold them, listening for their concerns.

It takes effort to keep your family intact; precious energy may be at a premium. Keep communicating openly during these challenging times. At the same time, talking with children about this can be tricky due to societal pressure and the difficulty of the situation itself. It will take some careful planning. Yet positive stories far outweigh negative ones.

> We not only told our children right away, but had them with us in the hospital to meet their baby sister. They touched her, held her, and even sang her songs. So sweet. No nightmares or problems at all. —A mom

> My two sons who are now older are kind of upset with us. They wish they would have pictures of them with their brother who died ten years ago when they were little. They can't get over that we "kept them away from him." I wish I could go back and do it over. —A dad

Not all parents are prepared to include their children in the early days of such a loss. Children can be very curious and needy, depending upon their age and personality style. If you feel you need to limit their awareness for a bit, be honest to a degree, holding back specific details until you feel ready and can be there for them. For example, one mother suggested that she "made a conscious choice to be low key with the children for almost a year." She told them that she was not feeling well and that there were personal things that she couldn't talk about right now. She promised them that she would fill them in when she felt better. At a later point, she told them more about how the baby had died and showed them some pictures of their brother. This worked for her and her family.

You will have to find what works for you. Look at your children's needs and personalities to decide if you think they are ready to hear the news. In the past when babies died, society did not promote openness, and children often did not know about siblings who died, many parents going to their graves with that knowledge. Surviving siblings were often surprised to discover this news later, when there was no opportunity to talk about it, leaving them in shock and sometimes even angry. Things have changed and there is more transparency and conversation about a baby's death. Don't hold back information for the sake of keeping secrets, since things come out much more these days. Whether the issue is the maturity of your children or your own unreadiness, take the time you need. But consider making a plan, or at least a commitment, to tell your children in the near future.

OPEN COMMUNICATION: GIVING THE NEWS

Ask your children what they have already heard. Clarify that information and determine what else needs to be discussed. Information should be based on your other children's age—toddlers may not understand details, but older children surely will. Generally, three to six year olds seem to be the most open, inquisitive, and amazing in their abilities to comfort their parents. Some parents think young children don't know what is going on and withhold information about what has happened. However, these children have vivid imaginations and when not told the real story will create their own story. This can become either a nightmare or a fairy tale, given that they don't have the entire story or are too young to understand it. If they are old enough, you can ask them directly; if they are young, it may come out at playtime.

> We asked our seven year old what she thought happened to the baby. We had decided not to be too graphic and explain our role at this time, so little had been said directly to her. She stated that the baby was really hurt and was not big enough to live, so it died. We added that it was a he, her brother, and that Simon had not been healthy from his little start in mommy's tummy. Nothing could have helped him get better. And she was right; he did die. She seemed satisfied and we felt that was good enough for now. Maybe someday when she is a woman, we will tell her more or maybe we won't. Don't have to worry about that now. —Anonymous

Our son was four at the time and [had] quite a great imagination. We started by asking him what he thinks happened to the baby. His reply was pretty typical, "Jonas was being chased by bad guys in mommy's tummy. One day he heard me say to my Power Ranger that I didn't really want to share my room with a new little boy, and he got mad. He beat the bad guy up and then just disappeared." We were floored. Where did that come from? So we explained that his story was very creative. However, Jonas was very, very sick and would never be able to eat or sleep or play with him. It was so sad when he died. We will miss him. —Anonymous

If your children are not very verbal or are young, you may wish to start conversations about the baby and what happened with play using stuffed animals, puppets, other toys, or by drawing. Things may flow from there. If it stalls, you might try another day. An example of how to use stuffed animals or a puppet to start a conversation is, "Polly the puppy is here to play. She loves to run and chase her tail. But today she is sad. Why is she sad do you think? Yes, her little brother died. I wonder why? She misses him and wants to lick his face. What should she do?"

Your children will watch how you handle this loss, even when you don't think they are. This impacts how they deal with it personally. They will respond to the loss of their baby sister or brother on a very personal level. Since most children behave as if they are the center of the universe, their responses usually revolve around how they see life (not just the loss) and the changes in their family. They may not be very understanding or patient about your needs or concerns, and you may not be as patient and understanding about theirs.

My children know that I was extremely ill and that their little brother was too weak to survive. The simple truth is often the best answer —Jennifer

Be careful about secrets and mixed messages. Many parents regret that they did not give enough thought about how to include their children and what to tell them given their ages and developmental stages. Many kids will wonder if they did something to cause it, so do give them a reasonable explanation as soon as you can. You don't want them imagining a series of explanations for what went wrong. You can adjust the storyline later if need be but some explanation for why the lights are low, why people keep coming, why you are home from work, and why the routine has changed is necessary.

Before you begin in-depth conversations with your children, first decide what you will tell others about the circumstances that brought you here, whether that means continuing the pregnancy or that the baby has died. What will your children think if you imply that the baby is fine and will be born in a few months but they hear about problems? And if you tell them that the baby died but others mention that you ended the pregnancy, they may ask if you killed the baby. Bluntness and simplicity just come out. You can count on your children hearing stories that are circulating. Be careful not to outright lie in order to protect them, as this can cause trust issues later on. But you may determine that some information need not be given at this time.

Sometimes parents tell the children one thing, such as, "The baby died suddenly and is in heaven," and family members another, such as, "We feel so guilty that we were the ones to choose the time and the manner of her death." If the children are old enough to hear the discrepancy between the two messages, they may get very confused. It might be better to tell them that explaining how and why the baby died to children their age is difficult. Promise to share more details when they are able to understand and reassure them that you love their sibling and did not want him or her to die. That way you are not lying or telling conflicting stories, but rather choosing not to tell the entire story for now. You may also choose to never tell the whole story to them, which is a decision you must make carefully. Be sure to keep your children's personalities and maturity levels in mind.

CHILDREN'S EXPERIENCES LIVING WITH THEIR PARENTS' LOSS

Your children experienced the death of their baby brother or sister and as a result they may feel less safe and secure. Their lives have changed abruptly and they may be confused about how to handle it. If they have not had pets die or other losses, they will need guidance about how your family handles it.

If you are listless and having trouble coping, you may wonder how you will take care of other children, both emotionally and physically. You may not have it together to fix meals, pack lunches, clean the house, and play with them. People may tell you to "get a grip" and "be there" for your children, but it is difficult to cope. How can you help someone else who is dependent upon you when you can't help yourself?

Some parents are able to give their living children plenty of attention, despite the struggles. It can bring comfort to you both. Others cannot find the strength to give anything to others, including their children. This is what happens with deep mourning, especially during the early days, weeks, and beyond.

As long as you, your partner, or parents ensure that your children are cared for, you should do what you need to do. You should not be judged for how you grieve. However, be confident that in time and with much grief work, you will find a new normal for yourself and your family. Getting there is not easy for most people, but it is possible. Use your faith, your family and friends, and all the resources you can find to be the parent of the child who may die or has died, as well as your living children. Seek help in getting to the place where you can cope and be the loving parent you wish to be.

Hopefully, your children will not have to witness a complete nervous breakdown, but it is unrealistic to expect children not to notice the sad atmosphere and the change in the household routine. You can explain that sometimes mommies and daddies get sad, too, and that crying makes us feel better sometimes, just like it does for them when they get a boo-boo or are scared or worried.

Many bereavement specialists encourage parents to be honest and involve their children in their journey. This can be a productive way to help the family to remain close and to learn to rebuild their life together.

When grief seems as if it is overwhelming you or if you feel so frustrated that you don't know what else to do, seek counseling. Getting outside help is necessary if you are depressed, thinking about or making suicide threats, self-harming, abusing substances, and/or harming others. It is best not to wait until it gets this bad. Seek help from counselors early in the grief process to help keep you and your children on track.

You will find many books for parents, families, and even teachers that discuss death as it relates to children. Depending on the child's age, there are many activities and ways to play with toys that help open up the conversation. A list of these resources can be found at the end of this book.

CHILDREN'S OWN EXPERIENCES

Children have different needs, and their responses will vary according to their age, their level of emotional awareness, and their personality. It helps to respond to them with these differences in mind. You know them best.

Young children often say things without much thought. Usually, they don't understand the consequences or impact. Their words and behaviors may touch you deeply, may be upsetting to you, or may be somewhere in between. Their questions may be direct, honest, and even repetitive. They may blurt things out at inopportune times and may tell others what they have heard. Most young children cannot keep secrets. Be patient and understanding.

As parents, you may try to protect your children from pain and sadness. Although this seems a worthy goal, the truth is, no matter how hard you try, you cannot protect them from such tragedies as having a sibling with challenges or who dies. Shielding them from trauma and deep loss is almost impossible and can lead you to feel like a failure when you see how strongly they are impacted by such loss. When they are in pain, naturally you are in pain; you can't kiss it away easily like a small wound, which only adds to your feelings of inadequacy and loss of control.

The most you can probably do is to hold, listen to, and comfort them while keeping them up to date on what is happening, appropriate to their age and maturity levels, of course.

Some Things That You Can Do

Listen to and answer your children's questions carefully, without too many words. They may really just want to know where the physical body is when they ask, "But where *is* he?"

Utilize resources such as *Healthy Mindsets for Super Kids* (Azri, 2013). This book teaches resiliency skills to children in a lighthearted way through games, worksheets, and comic books. The chapter on grief and loss for children might be something helpful to refer to now or later on. There are many, many other books that may be helpful, some of which are small and easy to read.

No one can predict how your children may react; learn about developmental stages so that you know how to respond as you comfort and communicate with each one.

Remember this is about them and the way they see the world. If you don't have the energy or time to "get in the puddle" with them to see through their eyes, find someone who does. This may be a good job for an aware grandparent, teacher, or aunt or uncle. You can get advice or help from a child development specialist or grief counselor.

If your children are in school, let their teacher and school counselor in on what has happened in a note or preferably a call. They can watch for signs, changes, and any difficulties.

A quick overview of common stages of development will be helpful. Keep in mind that these are only guidelines. Some children are wise beyond their years at age three, while older children seem babylike or unaware. You know your children best, so pay attention to how they respond to other life experiences and use your judgment as you attempt to understand and help them.

Do note that many children—of all ages—regress after a stressful event like this. Some examples are bedwetting, thumb sucking, tantrums, reduced language skills, and other signs of immaturity. This does not usually last, but it may be confusing to you, them, and those around them. Although not mentioned in every section below, regression is a normal behavior for children of many ages. Don't focus on that; allow your children to cope in the way that seems natural, unless you find it harmful to them or others. Awareness and patience are key.

CHILDREN AGED THREE YEARS AND YOUNGER

Children younger than three may not understand grief, death, or what is happening, but they sense that things have changed or that things are sad at the moment. They may also feel scared because children of this age have a strong need for routine and it is very likely that their routine has changed to some degree, even if temporarily. They also have a need for attention, such as hugs from their parents and reassurance, which may be difficult to give at the moment—or it might be exactly what you need to do right now.

Your young child may be reacting to the shift in the household and the lack of attention rather than to the prenatal diagnosis and pregnancy or death itself. Although this may be upsetting, remember that these are normal behaviors and something you cannot control. Very young children may not understand the meaning of "death" or "special needs." Some children do seem to relate to death and may make comparisons to their fish, the bug, or a bird that died in the yard. There are books that can guide you in helping children this age; there are even ones meant to be read aloud to them, especially for those children who are curious and ask questions. Some are listed in the resources at the end of this book.

> My daughter was only a year and a half old when our precious daughter Abigail passed away. She was at the hospital for Abigail's birth. When she came in to meet her sister she seemed very unsure, as everyone in the room was crying and very emotional, but I don't think she was old enough to understand what was happening.
> —Anonymous

> Emily was precocious for her young age of three. She sat on the bed holding Emmet, stroking his face, and kissing his cheeks and lips. Her questions were so profound and honest. Why did he have to die, when would she see him again, how would we deal with his room, and that she would miss playing with him, her "forever brother." How grateful we are that we included her. Now years later, she talks of that lovely time with him and seems to remember most of it.
> —Anonymous

Some Things That You Can Do

Give extra comfort to little ones; this may help calm them. If you are unavailable physically or emotionally, ask a grandparent or other close relative to help.

Offer reassurance to bring some calm and hope into the picture. Even children at this age know that something is not right, but they often don't have the words or capacity to deal with it on their own. You might say, "Things are different right now, but they will be okay soon." "Don't worry, honey, Mommy and Daddy love you." "The baby is not in pain. She still needs to stay in Mommy's tummy for a while and when she is born, you can see her and kiss her." "We all love your sister and will miss her."

Ask questions—simple ones—to determine how much your children understand and what they are thinking. Questions like, "Do you wonder what happened? So do we. If we learn more we will tell you." "Do you think that you or we did something wrong and that is why the baby is sick? That is not what happened." "Do you have any questions for mommy or daddy?"

Sand play, stuffed animals, puppetry, imaginary play, drawing, and finger painting can be useful in helping small children express feelings.

Don't overexplain. Listen to their words, musings, and questions. Keep your responses at their level. Don't go too deep unless your child is precocious and needs a deeper answer. A few sentences, after you clarify what they are asking, could be enough. Keep the door open for other questions or comments.

Never say that the baby "went to sleep" instead of "died." This could affect your children deeply. They may wonder if it could happen to them if they sleep. Though some words are hard to say, they need to be said. Don't let your sadness and fear keep you from honesty and openness.

Also, don't say that the baby was very sick and died, since that could scare small children the next time they—or other loved ones—have a cold, flu, or other illness. You could offer more information, saying something like, "When Grant was first made, it looks like he had some serious problems. We didn't know until recently that as he was growing these problems were getting worse. This doesn't happen to too many babies or people, and it didn't happen to you. But sadly, it did happen to our Granty."

CHILDREN AGED THREE TO SIX YEARS

Children in this age group still may not understand the permanency of death. Much of what was discussed in the previous section applies to children of this age. They may have some experience with a bird or pet that has died and might relate the baby's death to that experience. Offer these examples so that they have a story in common to talk about with you. Maybe a grandparent has died or someone else they knew. Comparing the similarities and differences might be a good way to begin the conversation. Speaking slowly, with a moderate amount of words, and listening to their questions while watching their behaviors will serve you well.

The idea of a baby sister or brother with special needs might be beyond their comprehension. However, if you can think of someone in the neighborhood, in school, or on television who has some challenges, this could be a good way to compare and contrast as they work to understand what might happen with their sibling.

> My two daughters were given a private tour of the hospital. They were given special pins, that they were big sisters of twins. They were allowed to ask questions and talk and [were] given straight answers by nurses and doctors who were sensitive to the fact that these girls were preparing for the death of one sister. —Lee

Many children of this age are curious and ask lots of innocent, powerful, and difficult questions. This may be traumatic for you or reassuring that they can be open and honest with you. They understand sadness and may want to fix it by offering solutions (sometimes profound solutions) that might even include magical thinking. They may share their tears freely. They hurt for you and themselves. They may even ask about whether their baby sister or brother was—or is—in pain. Depending upon their personality and level of shyness, it is possible that they will talk about their feelings and even their fears, especially if you make time for them and show some openness about what is happening.

Most children of this age group may wonder why their new baby brother or sister was born under those circumstances, and they may even think that they have done something wrong. It is common for children this age to also feel guilty, thinking that they (or you) may have done something to cause this. It is important to talk about this.

> My young niece recently suggested that maybe I did not eat right or take enough vitamins, therefore causing my son to die. Like most adults, she was looking for a rational answer about why a baby would die, assuming this doesn't just happen. —Sherokee

On the other hand, they may also believe that their sister or brother will come back and act like other children. They may talk of playing with their baby sibling either in your belly or at the cemetery, for instance. Some children like to bring toys, have conversations, and act out playful situations with their absent sibling who is clearly still present in their minds. Don't be worried about this. It happens all the time. One mom reported that her children played Ring Around the Rosie around the baby's headstone, an innocent game and a way to include their brother.

Children this age may not always understand the questions they ask, so rather than offer more complicated explanations than they can handle, seek clarification before answering. For example, "You say you want to know where baby Jenny is. What do you mean? Where is her body right now? Or where is she, meaning heaven or in our hearts? Tell me more about what you want to know." Or they may ask mom if she can hear them singing in mom's belly.

Some Things You Can Do

Listen carefully and clarify their questions.

Offer them quiet time to play with stuffed animals, puppets, or other items as they act out what is happening. This can be a very natural way for them to express their feelings and may show you what they are thinking.

Sit with them in the baby's room and talk about your hopes, their hopes, and any worries that they might have.

Feel free to ask if they feel bad that they—or perhaps someone else—could have caused this to happen. If you say it first, it might make it easier for them to speak about it out loud, too.

Be prepared for conversations about other loved ones who might die. In fact, it is very common for children this age to ask if you will die or if grandma will die?

Attention span is short, as are conversations. It shouldn't surprise you when they quickly move on to play, to ask about the puppy, or to whine for a cookie.

When we brought Lana home, our elder son was thrilled. To him, Down syndrome and spina bifida were sort of like a middle name and it was only much later that he grasped the meaning. —Lana's mom

"Mommy, are you going to die, too?" I replied, "Yes, it is true. In time, everyone dies. But hopefully it will be a very, very long time before that happens. I work hard to take good care of myself so I'll be here for years and years. And when that time does eventually come, I want you to know I will always be with you in your heart and looking out for you in Heaven." —Sherokee to her son Trevor, age four

CHILDREN AGED SIX TO NINE YEARS

Children in this age group most likely understand death and special needs to some extent, as they already may have experienced it in their everyday lives. Maybe a pet, relative, or neighbor died, or they have met people with special needs. Children of this age tend to need and accept a simplified explanation of death or disability; often a short and logical definition is enough. As with the previous age group, children ages six to nine may also ask difficult questions, although they may feel ambivalent about asking them. Many children in this age group, after experiencing death or being included in discussions about a sibling dying, may start to become fearful that their parents (or someone close to them) might die. This is a normal reaction to your family's loss.

You may find a child of this age comforting *you*. One eight-year-old boy climbed into bed with his mommy after she came home from the hospital without the baby. Few words were exchanged, but the message was clear. He was there for her and wanted to show his love. Watch for those opportunities and take advantage of them. This is a vulnerable time for children who want to help and understand but who are still developing and trying to figure life out.

Some Things You Can Do

Speak openly. Listen carefully. Answer questions truthfully but without extensive explanations unless they seem to need them.

Offer them jobs to do to help you or others.

Share resources that they can read at their level of understanding. Read with them and use this as a time for conversation.

Invite family members that they are close with to spend time with them. They may find it helpful to have conversations with others if it is too hard to have them with you.

Offer writing and drawing tools, clay, and other creative outlets so that they can express themselves.

Encourage them to spend some time with friends and play. This is something they need to do and will want to do, though they may feel guilty about leaving you or having fun when you are sad.

Keep communication lines open and check in fairly often but not necessarily every day.

CHILDREN AGED TEN YEARS AND OLDER

In this age group, children understand much about death and special needs, especially as they become older teens. They usually understand the concept that death is final and sometimes life is unpredictable. This can make it even harder, as they will be sad and show feelings at times. Then suddenly, they then may go on with their life, which is quite normal for most children, no matter their age. They may feel guilty (though not everyone does) for being able to have fun or to live their life when their sibling died or while you and others are so sad.

Children of this age might understand that everyone is not alike, and they may know children at school who have challenges. On the other hand, they are still self-centered children or teens and may not really understand or be patient when it comes to your need to focus on your pregnancy, your baby with special needs, or your feelings of grief and loss.

They may, however, have lots of questions about their own death and the afterlife, or they may need time alone to adjust to how their "normal" life has suddenly changed. Things are clearly different and they know it. You may see some regression and even anger and frustration about all the stress and emotions. They might be frustrated that no one will drive them to the mall or to their friend's house on their timetable. Maybe they resent the lack of attention they are getting and start behaving in sometimes destructive or defiant ways that generates interactions and responses from you.

Some Things You Can Do

Listen and ask open-ended questions. "What are you thinking about when we talk about Jaime?" "What is going on with you? You seem upset."

Be honest and open about what has happened and what difficulties, sadness, and frustrations you feel (in limited doses—don't overwhelm them with your problems).

Answer questions honestly without excessive explanation for their ages and maturity levels. They don't need to know about the other parents you have met and what problems their babies have or all the details the doctor has told you.

Allow them to escape to their room, to go outside to play, and time to be with their friends. They need breaks in more upbeat or playful places.

Share written resources to help them to better understand the baby's condition or what grief is all about.

Invite them to help with decision making and give them jobs so that they feel included. They could keep the list of places to visit and the things you are doing with your yet-to-be-born baby. Maybe they can be the journal keeper for these experiences. They could go shopping and pick out burial clothes or draw a picture or do graphic design for the baby's memorial service.

Show openness about other loss issues that they may be experiencing, such as the loss of a friendship, school-related problems, fears about people dying, and so on. This is a special time to create a bond and to talk about life's tough issues. Death is one of the big losses, but to a young person there are many other losses that impact them deeply.

Continue to say your baby's name out loud and tell older children why you are doing this. As a family, each person has a permanent place and each always will be loved and remembered.

Paige (age twelve) became even more rebellious than usual, fighting a lot with Stephen (her stepfather) and giving me a headache. She spent a lot of time with her brother in the hospital and did some very special things for him after the funeral. Since then, she has matured considerably and it seems that we are a lot closer. She has amazed me beyond belief. However, she is very careful with whom she shares her brother (his pictures and stories). She doesn't trust just anyone to confide in. —Anonymous

To summarize, children of all ages express different degrees of acceptance of this new situation. They will experience and express their grief and disappointment in unique ways. Some may show signs of regression, irritability, fears, inhibition, sleep or eating issues, while other children, especially older ones, may show anxiety and feelings of guilt. Some may be supportive and comfort you and other family members. Others may need to talk about their sibling's birth or death, as well as other things linked to the experience. They may feel bad about raising a painful topic with their parents and thereby purposely ignore their own emotional needs in order to protect their family. As parents, you may feel guilty, not only for your own emotions, but for those of your children. Since you can't stop them from feeling sadness and pain, your challenge is to offer a balance of support and openness about why pain is a natural way of showing love. You will all miss this baby if he or she dies. And you will have different dynamics in your family if the baby lives but has challenges. This is an ongoing loss without an end in sight. Although you may wish to share some things but not others, it is not wise to protect your children from the basic realities of the situation by keeping secrets. Many parents have tried this and learned the hard way how unhelpful and even harmful it can be.

SOME THINGS YOU CAN DO

Use the appropriate words, though they are hard to say. Don't use euphemisms or fabricate a nicer ending than the actual one. For example, you could say something like, "We are so sad to tell you that our sweet baby has some serious problems. She may not live after she is born. This is a terrible surprise and very sad. We will get through this together." Or, "Our little munchkin had serious problems and has died. We are all going to be sad for a long time."

Avoid the words "gone to sleep" or "gone away" since children may worry that they—or someone they love such as mom, dad, or other siblings—could also "go away," never to return. This causes confusion and should be avoided. Explain in simple words that your baby has a certain condition, which means that his or her body cannot survive. Reassure them that this is not something that could happen to them or to you.

It is best to be truthful, while also taking into consideration your child's age. Simplify the truth or keep it to a minimum. In the long term, be honest with your children, which reinforces trust, respect, and understanding. Assist them in grieving the loss of their sibling *with* you. As they grieve, they will also heal with time, a priceless gift you can give them by helping them to understand what is happening.

Allow them to talk about their concerns, your pregnancy, and the loss. Most people benefit from talking about their emotions. Help them debrief and reframe the trauma. Encourage difficult questions, allowing the time and space to be emotional without feeling guilt.

Tell your children how much you love them. Take the time to let them know that you are okay but may need some time before you feel better. Don't be afraid to show some raw feelings to your children. It may help them to feel normal and to understand empathy better. They can come to see that things can get better with time.

If your baby will be born with special needs, inform your children about the baby's condition. If possible, perhaps you can talk about the things that you believe or hope that he or she will be able to do. Be as positive as you can be given the circumstances.

If your baby dies, invite your children to be involved in some way. They could do a reading at the service, help dig the grave, or write a poem or song.

21

WORKPLACE ISSUES

Soon after a baby dies, the realities of life drop into your lap. Suddenly, it seems, you may be faced with the ordinary life decision about going back to work. Both mom and dad may have this issue, which will need to be addressed.

Returning to work or not, telling people what happened, getting support for both partners, and deciding on your focus as you move forward are but a few of the common work challenges felt by others who have been down this road. If you are staying home, feel free to skip this chapter and move on.

BACK TO WORK?

When and whether you go back to work is a personal decision that will depend upon your physical and emotional health, your healing needs, your finances and family needs, the policies and politics of your workplace, and, perhaps, the laws of your country. Whether you decide to go back to work soon after a loss or down the road, how you deal with the people at work, and if you can do your work are worth serious planning and consideration.

> I needed to get back to work as soon as possible. It was a bit of a safe haven, a place where I could be busy and not be overcome by my sad thoughts each and every hour of the day. At least I got a break from the "dark life" I was now destined to live. —Anonymous

I had no choice. Due to my line of work and our small company, I was back on the job within five days. It was hard to navigate the two parts of myself. I wanted to be at home with my wife, giving her comfort and laying around the house for a while. We had things to organize so we could get back on our game. Instead, I was in a job that no longer mattered. I was expected to keep up my quota and get back on track as if we never had the baby. Talking with my boss did not change things. Due to finances and my fear about how I would support my family, I had to tough it out. Not sure how I lasted two more years, but I did. —A dad

TAKING A LEAVE FROM WORK

Since each country, state, and even each company has its own laws and policies about time off, disability, and parental leave, it is impossible to be very specific about what options you may have. For example, in Australia, parental leave is paid for women after the birth of a registered stillbirth (up to fourteen weeks of paid leave); after a pregnancy termination, paid leave may be negotiated. Currently in the United States, there are no specific laws that give grieving parents more than a few days off. Although some groups are working to add to Family Medical Leave Act (FMLA), at this time each company and workplace sets the policy. You or an advocate should contact your manager and the human resources department to ask about your options. There are a number of managers, owners, and companies who will make exceptions when there is no official leave policy in place for people in your situation. They may be able to pay you for the leave time, they might be willing to give you time off without pay, or they may allow you to work part time. They may even allow late starts or extra break time during the day, if you find it difficult to get to work or remain focused. If your job has any dangerous components to it (such as heavy or sensitive equipment, driving, or patient care), you may need to carefully assess whether you are ready and able to return immediately.

When working to obtain more time off or increased flexibility, you may need to make the case that a death is a death. And in this situation—and for mom especially—it also includes a birth, which deserves recovery time. The age of the loved one or the size of the body should not make a difference. If you were expecting to welcome a baby into your home and now she or he has died, you will grieve and mourn. Period. Two weeks is not enough time to do the hard work of healing, which unfolds over a lifetime. The most intense grief can last for many months or longer.

How you present your story and your request may be important, especially if you feel you are totally at the mercy of your employer. Be respectful of their position if you can. They are without an employee who contributed and who is needed. They may have difficulty finding funds to pay both you and a replacement. If you are gone, is there someone else who can do your work without it becoming a terrible burden? How long will it take to train someone to do your job? Given all of that, you may be able to take a leave either with or without pay.

> My assistant had a loss. It was so sad. I did my best to be supportive, understanding, and compassionate. I even bought her flowers and gave her coupons to restaurants every week for a while. Even after a few months I began to notice that she was making mistakes, sending out the wrong data, and losing things. She didn't come in as often as needed (I gave her flexible hours) and was clearly in a fog. I had no one else; what was I to do? I kept hoping she would find a new normalcy and be more on top of things soon. But what if it took as long as grief can take? I can't afford to lose money, pay for poor work, and hire someone else to cover her. And I don't want to appear to be a heartless boss. What is a manager or owner supposed to do in this situation? Even when our employees come first, we are torn about how it impacts the company, too. —Anonymous

RETURNING TO WORK

Before you return to work, it is important to help set the tone to welcome you back. Do you want people to know all or some of what happened? Do you want them to acknowledge your loss? Do you prefer to talk with each person individually or do you wish to have everyone hear the story at once? Are you okay with your manager or boss telling what she or he knows or do you want it told in your words? Keep in mind that if someone else tells the news, it may be a bit like the telephone game. They could use words and explanations that are not quite accurate. In that case, you might have to retell people anyway.

Most managers and colleagues are not well prepared for your return. They may not know what happened and what you might need upon return. Without proper preparation and guidance, you can expect a number of responses, ranging from coworkers asking you to repeat the story (over and over) or silence because they are hesitant to ask you questions. They do not want to hurt you. These people are waiting for you to tell them more. Or they respect that you don't want them to know, so they won't ask, even if you wish that they would. If you prepare them ahead of time, you can feel assured that everyone got the news, which saves you from retelling the story. When they hear it from you, or an advocate, the story should be the same for everyone. Think about what might work best for you. If you take some control here, it may help reduce the discomfort of your coworkers, who are usually at a loss as to how to behave around you.

Many parents have reported that telling the news prior to returning helped them immensely. Hilary wrote letters for her principal to read to the teachers and to her class prior to returning after her baby Natalie died. She found it easier to face going back because she was comfortable that they had the news along with her suggestions on how to help.

James asked to meet with his team at work to explain what happened and to offer suggestions about how to proceed once he returned. Jillian asked an advocate to meet with her supervisor and her entire unit to inform them and to prepare them for specific ways to welcome her back, such as saying her baby's name out loud. She even explained that Jillian would have a picture of her baby on her desk and she didn't want people to freak out. She then offered some guidance about how to view the picture of a child who is dead (but well loved).

You may choose to tell coworkers ahead of time in a meeting, a call, an e-mail, or a letter, or you may wait until your return. You may ask a manager or human resources professional to relay the circumstances to the rest of the team. In any case, what you say to them is a personal decision. In the United States, you are protected by the Health Insurance Portability and Accountability Act (HIPAA) privacy rule, which protects your privacy as a patient, and you may not have to disclose any of the circumstances surrounding your medical absence. Of course, because pregnancy is somewhat public at some point and because you are likely on friendly terms with coworkers, you may feel compelled to address that your baby did not make it. What and how much you decide to tell your coworkers and supervisors are up to you.

You may worry that people will judge you or not understand. They might think that this impacts your work environment and relationships. Let's be honest; that can happen. Because it is difficult to be judged and to go forward in a normal kind of way, you may wish to choose your words carefully. You may even want to tell only part of the story, perhaps saying that the baby was stillborn. Just be sure to be consistent and don't tell some coworkers one thing and the others another. Secrets rarely remain secrets. How will it impact you and your work if you have different stories circulating? This is why putting what happened in writing for everyone to see may help you to stay consistent. In the end, it is about you and what you need to say and about how you feel about what has happened.

Some examples of how others announced their losses to their coworkers follow.

- "Our baby died. We are heartsick. I do want to talk about Lilly but not about how she died. It is too painful [or too sad], but she is, and always will be, our beloved first daughter."
- "Liam is gone and it is very hard to live without him. He will always be my baby and I welcome talking about him at work during breaks [or whenever you prefer]. He is a huge part of our family and my life, so please know that I will need your patience and understanding as I try to pick up the pieces getting to my new normal. Since Liam is our beloved son who happens to have died way too soon, you can expect to hear me talk about him and share the memories I do have. As his parent, I will be learning how to actively parent him in my heart and spirit."
- "Right now I prefer to focus on my job, so I hope that you can be supportive by doing [or not doing] the following [for example, saying his name, asking me how my partner and I are doing, remembering him and us on holidays and special times, donating to a special baby loss charity, etc.] during break time but not during work time."
- "Sometimes breathing is even difficult, so please allow me to have my difficult times. Loving someone so much means we miss her deeply every minute of every day. I am doing what I can to get

through this, but I will never get over her. Thank you for caring [or asking]."

FULL OR PART TIME?

Will you go back to full time or is part time an option? Think about realistic options before discussing it with your boss. If you feel you must or are required to work full time, ask your manager if you can have some flexibility on those days when it is difficult to leave the house or to concentrate for the entire day. This can go a long way toward reducing your stress and making you a better employee. There will be some days that are tough to navigate and you may need a place to hide out or a chance to go home early. Have a frank conversation with your manager ahead of time or on your first day back so that you both can be honest about what is needed from you and what you are able to give. Maybe you can work from home a bit, starting part time and working up to full time, or perhaps you can negotiate some other agreed-upon option.

Don't be surprised if your feelings about your work have changed. Your life has changed, your perspective is different, and your mind may not be able to concentrate on something that now seems unimportant. This is very common and understandable. You may be absorbed by thoughts of your baby and by what your home and work life should have been. Navigating these choppy waters often requires help from counselors, human resources, local or online support groups, spiritual leaders, and good friends. You need to adjust as you find that "new normal." That will take time and it won't be easy. But it is possible and many have done it. In some cases, parents needed to make changes in their positions at work; in others, they changed jobs or careers in order to go forward in a positive and different direction. Still others found it hard to think about another place to work because they were so well loved and supported during this difficult time in their lives.

It is common for people at work and in the neighborhood to ask dad, "How is your wife doing?" They often don't ask how dad is doing, which is unfortunate. If you are asked how your wife is doing, consider one dad's answer, "Physically she is recovering well; emotionally we are both a wreck. This has been hard on us and will not be easy for a long time, if ever. Thank you for asking."

Another dad shares this, "I am different. Not the guy you used to know. Our world has turned upside down. Have patience with me if I show my anger, frustration, or am distant. I am coping in the best way I know how right now."

FINDING A NEW FOCUS

It is very common for parents to come to the conclusion that they can no longer be at their workplace. Sometimes the empathy and flexibility wanes and you may feel you are expected to be back to "normal" or at your previous production levels, yet this doesn't seem possible.

Some parents report that they don't feel understood and supported after the loss of their baby, as if he or she was insignificant. You might feel angry and frustrated at coworkers or about supervisors' comments or silence about your baby. Sometimes it is too difficult when everyone knows both the "old you" and the changing or "new you." You may need a fresh start. Although these feelings are common, quitting work outright may not be the best thing for you to do for yourself or for your family. Think it through carefully, talk with others, and explore how this could work. What you don't need now is another stressor in your life. Maybe you'll need to tough it out for a bit until you develop another plan of action. Before acting, do take some time to think about it. If your financial situation requires your income or if you will be isolating yourself from a supportive, social network, exhaust all other options before quitting.

Sadly, there are plenty of people who feel misunderstood and unsupported at work. You may find that management or even fellow employees expect you to be back to normal after a week or two. This is not usually possible for most people. It may be worth it to give it your all for a while to see if you can make things work out.

If you find it too painful or too stressful to stay, you may choose to ask for a leave without pay or to quit outright. If you decide that you just can't go back and want to quit or take a long leave, ask yourself a few practical questions. Put them in writing and look carefully at your answers, as this may help guide you. Some things to consider: Will it really help not to have some of my close colleagues near me each day? What could I do instead? What are my options? Should I look for a job before

I quit? Can I afford to not work for a while? Could I work from home for some time, minimizing the tension I feel from others at work? In the end, do what you need to do. Maybe you need more time at home. Maybe you will be ready to look for other work in the future.

Natalie worked in a mental health clinic as a support assistant. After her baby died at term, she reported that these supposedly caring therapists and staff members didn't reach out to her with well wishes during her leave of absence. She felt hurt and abandoned by the very people who should know better. When she returned to work, not a word was said and no genuine acknowledgment or compassion was offered. Her coworkers had left most of her work piling up on her desk. It hurt her deeply and it still did years later. During the first few weeks she tried to make it work, but the burden and the added pain from coworkers was stressful. Even though she needed the job to support her children, she soon quit. She did not regret it. Clearly, she did not belong where her and her family's loss meant so little.

> I could not go back to consulting work, where I once stood and faced others with confidence and knowledge. I realized I had no confidence left and I did not have the energy to even talk with human resources to set up more communication workshops. So I left that world and began to substitute teach. Some days I made myself unavailable so I could just stay in bed or at home. It worked out better. Now, years later, I wish I had stayed at it; I loved the work and it was good money. But at the time, it didn't seem possible. —Sherokee

Give yourself grace as you attempt to integrate back into society after suffering such a loss. People have done this throughout the ages, and there is clearly no single "right" way to do it. Find your way; adjust as you learn what works for you. Believe in yourself and your ability to adapt and grow while loving and remembering your baby.

TIPS AND ADVICE

- Consider your legal, financial, and social options. Are you able to return to work? Can you afford to not return to work? What alternatives are available?

- Speak to your human resources department to find out about employee assistance programs (for example, gradually returning to work, transferring to a different department, counseling, etc.).
- Prepare yourself before returning to work. Do you want others to know? Would you rather not? Make mental notes of how you would like to handle others in the workplace.
- If you have been gone a long time due to your pregnancy, mom, it may be especially awkward to go back. If you haven't kept in touch during the ensuing months, putting something in writing explaining what you want your coworkers to know and what they can do when you return is a good idea.
- Seek support outside work. This will make it easier for you if you're not up to your usual work standards and feeling anxious about repercussions. This way you will be able to be honest about your work struggle without consequences.
- Join a support group. As we have reminded you throughout this book, speaking to those who have walked the walk will provide you with practical and emotional insights into navigating this very difficult time in your life.
- Find support online. Before you begin posting on a group, look back over the previous posts. You will get a feel for the members. Are they whiners and complainers who use social media to spout off but don't really want help or support? Or are they kindhearted people who have been there and truly show their care and concern to those who are hurting? If you don't feel comfortable and don't like the tone of conversation, keep looking. You will find a better option.

22

POSTPARTUM AND SELF-CARE

As a mother who has most of the same needs as mothers with living babies, you will experience postnatal symptoms during the postpartum period, even though your baby has died. It is estimated that 10 to 15 percent of all new mothers experience postpartum depression. It may be higher for moms who have a special needs child or a baby who has died.

The postpartum period generally lasts about six to eight weeks. It is common to feel that you do not have the right to have postpartum symptoms if your baby died. Some of the symptoms are fatigue, sadness, hopelessness, changes in appetite or sleep, confusion, intense crying, feelings of wanting to escape, and more. Of course, these are also signs of grief, so it may be hard to determine exactly why you feel the way you do. Seek help and guidance if you think you may have postpartum depression.

You may feel deeply preoccupied with thoughts of your baby, which can last a long time. This is totally normal. You would be very busy with your baby if she had lived. You probably would have had little time for anything else. If you don't have other children at home, you may wonder what to do with your time. You may need to fill your time with thoughts of your baby and projects that honor her and help others. Of course, if your baby is alive with a limited lifespan or abilities, you may also have postpartum depression symptoms and the added complication of providing care when you have little energy.

The quotes from other mothers in this book may help you to feel less crazy and less alone, and the resources we share may offer support and guidance about taking care of yourself and when to seek help. Caring for yourself at this time is important but not always easy to do. Put some of your energy into your own healing. No one can do this but you.

TAKE CARE OF YOURSELF

Although taking care of yourself may be the last thing on your mind, it is important for you and your family. If you think having another baby may be in your near future, it is also important to regain your emotional and physical health. However, during the early days, many mothers talk about wanting to die or to go to sleep to escape. Of course, this makes sense. You can't easily stop thinking about the significant loss that has altered your life completely. You may feel you can't live your life without your baby. We know. We have been there.

> Being at home without a baby and facing his room that we never finished just got to me. I sobbed and sobbed. Eating, sleeping, even breathing didn't really matter. I just wanted my arms filled with my son. —Emma

> It seemed so unfair. I wanted a baby, not postpartum depression and empty arms. I was exhausted. It seems like I wandered around all day sighing and rubbing my nose with harsh tissue. At my follow-up visit, my doctor talked about hormonal changes that, when combined with the normal response of grief, can be very overwhelming. I am glad she said that. At least I knew some of it would get better. —A mom

Bleeding and Pain

You may have some heavy bleeding and some pain, which can result from cramps, stitches, bruising, or surgery if you had a caesarean. Hopefully, you were given advice and literature on wound care and how to deal with your pain before leaving the hospital. If you did not, call your clinic or doctor immediately. If you have never recovered from birth before, you may need to do some reading or talk with your provider. You may need some pain relief; don't be afraid to ask for it. Also learn the signs to watch for that could necessitate a trip in to the clinic or office, such as fever, abnormal discharge, swelling, odor, or abnormal tenderness. Don't overdo it in the first weeks following the birth, and longer if you had a C-section.

Breast Care and Milk

You may be surprised that your breasts produce milk and engorge, even if your loss was early in pregnancy. Your body knows what to do when you have a baby, even in this situation. However, it may seem like a slap in the face as it reminds you that you should be either still pregnant or nursing a baby. Some mothers say that they were given no information about this and were deeply surprised. This is a normal part of the process after a baby is born, whether she lives or dies. Expect tenderness and swelling or pressure. Lactation consultants disagree about how to deal with swollen breasts and whether to express a small amount of milk for comfort. Speak with your provider about what has worked for other mothers. *Mother Care* (Ilse, Anderson, and Funk) is a small booklet about self-care after a birth, procedure, and loss. You may find other birth books that address this.

You may be offered medication that will make the milk "dry up"; however, because it has been associated with adverse effects, many doctors prefer mothers to wear a tight bra and allow the milk to dry up naturally over several days. This can be painful, so you may try expressing a bit for relief. Discuss options for relief with your provider.

More mothers have asked about milk donation after a loss. Since the breasts are making milk and there is often a need to make something positive out of this tragic experience, you may be interested in considering this idea. You'll need to find out if you are a good candidate, as the milk must be appropriate for preemie babies. If you are able to donate milk, you would need to pump and keep the milk flowing for a while. There is often a need for milk for babies who are in the neonatal intensive care unit or who need donated milk for other reasons. Ask for help finding a local milk bank (or one that will accept your milk despite being far away). The Human Milk Banking Association of North America (www.hmbana.org), the Australian Breastfeeding Association (www.breastfeeding.asn.au), or the European Milk Banking Association (www.europeanmilkbanking.com) might be options. You or your care provider may even find more options. Mothers who have donated their milk report a sense of satisfaction that they can find something positive in the darkness of their loss. Milk donation is a potential option for some, though sometimes milk cannot be accepted, for example, due to illness or infection.

General Fatigue and Feelings of Grief

You may feel fatigued and sleep, which is an understandable response in your situation. You were pregnant, had a birth or horrible procedure, and now are living without your baby in your arms. Such emotional turmoil combined with the hormonal changes explains it. Some other feelings you may have can include tearfulness, anxiety, disturbed sleep, forgetfulness, confusion, deep sadness, and poor concentration, to name a few. Rest is important to help you regain strength and reduce these symptoms. Support from others is very helpful. Let your feelings out in some manner (crying, hitting a pillow, creating something, sharing them with others, etc.) rather than holding them in. You could write; listen to or create music; join a support group, in person or online; or find other creative outlets through the arts. Social media and the Internet are ways to connect with others. You could also work with nonprofits, which are always seeking volunteer support.

A common message understood by therapists all too well is that grief can be delayed but not denied. The healthy way to deal with such a serious loss is to face it and go through it, not around it. If not, it will eventually catch up to you, resulting in less-healthy consequences down the road. Make time for yourself and your healing. Sleep when you can or at least lay down and rest if you can't sleep. Remember that feeling tired and overwhelmed after having a baby is normal. You can read much more on healthy grieving in chapter 23, "Grief and Healing."

Postnatal Depression or Grief?

Postnatal depression affects some mothers. The behaviors and feelings of grief can look like severe depression. Some of the symptoms of grief include hopelessness, tearfulness, irritability, listlessness, and irrational fears. Extensive time in bed, anxiety about returning to work, confusion, extreme fatigue, sleeplessness, continual sighing, and disinterest in life are very common both in grief and depression. This baby is gone and your hopes for the future have been dashed. The sadness and shock may feel intense and last for a long while. When you love someone this much, you will grieve deeply for months and years. Though the intensity reduces over time, it never totally goes away for most mothers and fathers. This does not mean you are clinically depressed.

There are medical providers who prescribe medication to reduce the natural symptoms of grief. Although postpartum depression affects about 10 to 15 percent of women, it is commonly accepted that not all moms require medication or treatment for their symptoms. Instead, they need understanding and advice about how to grieve in a healthy manner. No one can say for sure what will work best for you. There are natural means that can be explored before resorting to medication, but there is no medication for grief that can take the pain away. Most experts suggest that doing grief work is the best medicine to mend a broken heart. However, your doctor may believe that you need medication, so you probably should hear why he or she feels it is the best option for you. It is possible that you may wish to follow his or her professional and expert advice. However, if you do not agree, you could read more about how to help yourself and get another opinion from another doctor. In the end, it is between you, your partner (if you have one), and your medical provider.

> I had never taken medication before. I couldn't believe my doctor prescribed it without even talking with me about what I was going through. I feel like there are other things I can try first. I wish I would have had a better conversation before leaving. —A mom

If you have had mental health issues previously or you feel that you don't know how to cope, it is wise to get help from professionals. Getting references is a good idea, as there are therapists who are familiar with infant loss and special needs children and others who are not.

> We went to see someone and he was so off base we had to leave. His view of baby loss was disrespectful. He kept talking about the trauma of me quitting my job and that our financial situation must be stressing us out. —A mom

There are some mothers who develop seriously destructive thoughts or even hallucinations after a baby dies. Talk with someone to help you to distinguish normal feelings of grief from clinical mental health issues. If symptoms persist, talk with your provider, especially if you have active thoughts of hurting yourself or someone else. This is serious and you need help if it comes to this.

COPING

How you cope and move forward relates to how you take care of yourself. If you don't want to be sick or become unhealthy, you need to take care of yourself. You will feel better and more able to deal with the changes and challenges in your life.

Prioritize caring for yourself, though it may seem hard to do that right now. If you are to heal and become healthy again, doing some important and basic things is vital. If you hope for another pregnancy in the near future, it is even more important to get your body and your mind ready.

Professionals who study grief recovery recommend the following five steps: seek support, drink fluids, eat healthy, exercise, and sleep well in order to regain health more quickly. Keep in mind that this does not mean that you give up your motherhood or that you will stop hurting or stop remembering your baby. It just means that you can get your body and mind into more healthful state by following the advice provided in the next section.

TIPS AND ADVICE

- Seek support, especially from those who understand. To find help, contact your hospital social worker, your clergy or doctor, or look online for support groups, counselors, organizations, and reliable websites that help you get in touch with people who understand and can be supportive.
- Drink fluids, preferably water, throughout the day. Avoid caffeine if possible, since it causes dehydration, which means you need to drink

about eight more glasses of water for each cup of coffee or caffeinated tea. Do this especially during the early days after your loss.

- Eat healthy foods and limit sugar, especially processed sugar.
- Exercise each day—bounce on a mini trampoline, which can boost your immune system, jog, walk, or take classes. The endorphins help you feel better after exercise.
- Sleep, or at least rest, each night to the best of your ability. Keep a notebook and pen nearby to capture important thoughts. Then visualize yourself in a calm and peaceful place where sleep might come more easily.
- Think positive thoughts when you can, pray for peace, guidance, and love, and believe that you can make it through this difficult time.

> Additionally, lavender aromatherapy is very helpful in producing a calming effect and it will also help you sleep. There are other essential oils that produce relaxing, sedating and antianxiety benefits such as bergamot (relaxing), mandarin (calming), jasmine (sedating), and sandalwood (sedating). —Dr. Ivy Margulies, clinical psychologist and death midwife

- Make time for yourself, even if you have other children at home. You can reflect, meditate, write, daydream, or sit in the sun. Reflect on yourself, think about your baby, read or exercise, or do nothing at all.
- Writing is helpful for many people. Find a healthy way to get your emotions out. Whether you have feelings of fear, hopelessness, guilt, anger, shame, hope, or gratefulness, put those emotions on paper. Someday you might find the writings enlightening, when you see how you changed and even grew over time.
- It's okay to cry but be sure you have soft tissues. It is okay to allow yourself to be miserable. You have recently given birth after devastating news and your hormones are raging. It is normal to feel a wide range of emotions, and there is nothing wrong with needing time to process them.
- Find a support group to join. Many parents are grateful for their support groups. Whether you join a group for women who have received a poor or fatal prenatal prognosis or any other type of group, you may appreciate the mutual exchange. When you hear other's stories and tips, you'll come to see that you are not alone. You may

make some good friends there. You'll find some support groups in the resources at the end of this book.

- Advocate for your needs. Others can only guess what might help you. Speak up and find your voice if you can.
- There are some things you can do that will take your mind to more healing places, using different parts of your brain. Yoga, interacting with pets, riding horses, making and listening to music, and praying and meditating are a few ideas.

> I felt less alone and more understood after attending a group for parents who terminated. We didn't judge each other. I felt safe and yet so sad. We cried a lot and now I have some new friends.
> —Isabelle

- Seek a healthy lifestyle. If you find this hard to do alone, find a friend or trainer to help keep you on track. Or keep a diet and fitness journal. Ask your partner or parent to help you set up a plan and invite them to support you each week.
- Seek professional support. Sometimes even with the best self-care methods, you may develop depression, anxiety, relationship issues, or even posttraumatic stress symptoms. As moms, we sometimes feel that we must keep it together for the family. However, it is vital to speak to someone if you feel like things are not quite right. You could start by talking to a friend, family member, or support group pal. If you think it is serious, find a professional counselor, clinical social worker, or psychologist. There are many clinicians who have experience working with women in your situation and who will assist you with your feelings. There are many trials in your relationships and within your own head. Talk it through with someone who understands and can offer advice.
- You may find it difficult to believe that you will smile, laugh, or have hope again. Yet it can happen. Your view of life may change—oftentimes for the better—as you realize that people, life, and love are so important. You may discover that you don't sweat the small things and may have little patience for others who whine and complain all the time. Changes may evolve slowly, but changes do, and can, come. Stay healthy, take care of yourself, and ask others to help you accomplish this in an effort to find a better tomorrow. Remember, you are a parent and no one can take that from you.

23

GRIEF AND HEALING

Why do you have to spend time learning about grieving when you want to spend time parenting your beloved baby? There is nothing right or fair about this. You may feel resentful and deeply upset that you are here and not there. Your world is under water and dreams are destroyed. Such a deep loss brings reminders of how much you love your baby. That depth of love naturally is followed by the normal need to grieve after such a loss. According to Vicki Culling in *Holding on and Letting Go*, "Love always leads to feelings of grief, and the complexity of the bond we hold with our child is expressed in the complexity of our grief."

Parents who share their stories in this book say they felt like they had been sucked into a vortex of darkness and pain. This club, as some people describe it—the club you never wanted to join and paid the highest price in order to become a member—is a shocking place to find yourself. You may feel thrown into a world you assumed belonged only to others. What should have been one of the happiest moments of your life turned into a shattered dream, a nightmare that just has to end. But doesn't.

In order for you—and for your friends and family—to make sense of the intense feelings that follow the news of your prenatal diagnosis or the loss of your perfect baby, you must understand that important connections, designed to build attachment between mother and child, occur before the birth of the baby. According to Kennel and Klaus's "pregnancy attachment theory" (1976), the attachment of the baby to mom and dad occurs through

- planning the pregnancy,
- confirming the pregnancy,
- accepting the pregnancy,
- feeling fetal movement,
- accepting the baby as a person,
- giving birth,
- hearing and seeing the baby,
- touching and holding the baby, and
- caring for the baby

We would add that playing house as a child is probably the beginning of the attachment process. You will notice that most of the list above occurs well before the birth of the baby, which can help you understand why there is significant grief when a baby dies of any gestation or age and why deep sadness and grief results from the loss of the dream of a perfect baby or when there are serious disabilities. Although many would have you believe that there is no attachment to a baby who is not yet born, that is not the truth. Experiencing a prenatal diagnosis or a pregnancy loss is a very sad and traumatic experience that is life altering for the baby and the entire family.

> I was in complete shock when I found out that my baby wasn't going to live. I remember lying on that table and looking at Gabriel on the monitor and wondering "what can we do to fix it?" but the doctor was trying to tell us that there was nothing we could do. —Anonymous

> Being told that our daughter would be born with spina bifida and very probably Down syndrome meant a lifetime of care, special needs, and being looked at by other people. Although we should have not cared about others' opinions, in the first few days we felt like failures and felt our child would be a burden. It was hard to see beyond our pain. —Lana's mom

GRIEF HURTS

Why does it hurt so much when you get this news and make this decision to either continue or end the pregnancy of your loved baby? Grief is hard work and can take a lot of time. It is intense, ongoing, overwhelming at times, and necessary in order to heal. Note, we did not say "recover" or "forget," but "heal" while keeping your child in your heart for the rest of your life. People experience grief in different ways. The mourning process—the actions that result from the feelings of grief—is unique, yet it connects you with others who have grieved throughout time. The feelings and needs experienced by most loved ones left behind are universal.

You may experience grief as sadness, weeping, and anguish in missing your baby. Additionally, there are physical signs such as shortness of breath, heart palpitations, stomach upsets, and various other aches and pains. Overall, we know that intense pain and grief can last for months and even years. Very few people actually ever "get over" the loss of a loved one, including a baby (as if they should!). Someone special will always be missing and he will always be a beloved family member held closely in your heart. Although people suggest that you can recover from grief (and they often want you to do so quickly), it is more accurate to say that you can heal, but you'll always remember and experience times of sorrow and hopefully some joy. As one father said, "The wound heals, but the scar never goes away."

Many mothers describe feelings of grief and sadness while their child is still alive in the womb. This can be called "anticipatory grief" or "early grief." If you felt your baby move but knew something was terribly wrong, it must have been difficult when others viewed your pregnancy as normal. Knowing the hope and joy would come to an end, it must have been challenging. You probably had bittersweet feelings about the progression of the pregnancy, perhaps not wanting it to end so that you could still *be* with your baby, who was still safe within your womb.

Deep anguish is often expressed by wailing, sighs, shortness of breath, sobbing, or continuous crying. The tape in your head keeps rewinding and you may keep trying to rewrite the script. It should have ended differently. The feeling of empty arms and a broken heart are common if your baby died. Your arms should be filled; sometimes a doll or teddy bear provides a brief sense of relief. The ache is persistent and words seem empty. You may wonder how you will endure or even how you will continue to live. These feelings exist for the loss of healthy babies, as well. As time goes on, feelings of grief and loss will grow for a while and may include

- Emotional feelings of sadness, anger, fear, depression, confusion, dismay, loneliness, and love
- Preoccupation with thoughts about the baby, fantasies, and fear of going crazy
- Physical signs such as aches, emptiness, lack of strength, heart palpitations, nausea, stomach pain, phantom baby kicks, head-aches, dry mouth, and plenty of sighing
- Social symptoms such as a desire to be left alone, problems com-municating, difficulty planning the future, relationship issues, dis-interest in your other children, and lack of concern about work or your home

TYPES OF LOSSES

When your baby dies—or the loss of the dream of a perfect baby oc-curs—it is viewed in the counseling world as a *primary loss*. In other words, a significant loss. You also experience multiple secondary losses such as the loss of ideals, loss of hope, loss of dreams, loss of family, loss of innocence, and loss of security and safety, to name just a few. This adds up to a pile of sadness and pain. Viewed both internally and exter-nally, you and others may wonder how someone survives this. Yet virtu-ally all bereaved parents do somehow. The early days are especially hard.

> I went home feeling very ill; I had this feeling of being on a roller coaster that would never stop. And I felt so alone, as though my life had ended, and I couldn't really verbalize why. —Stephanie

HONORING YOUR BABY AND EXPRESSING YOUR GRIEF

For decades, women and their families were told that they should "overcome" or "recover" from their losses. They needed to "cease bonds" with their precious children and focus on a *new* future. Thankfully, we now know that this is neither helpful nor possible. This lifelong process begins with deep anguish for all involved. As it progresses, there are many things you can do to honor your dream and the perfect baby you sought. You will find your own ways to express your inner feelings so that they don't overwhelm or overtake you. And you may want to find meaning as you work toward accepting that the loss is real and that your baby is not coming back. You'll probably find the love and the joy you had for your baby and maybe you will even create legacies for her. Remember that you will always be the parent of this child. As you continue these bonds, you create new memories. You can organize annual events or work with a charity in memory of your baby. You can even join others or make donations to help find cures for the problems your child had.

As you adjust over time to your loss, you may find that you become a better person or notice the importance of the relationships in your life. Tragedy can result in beautiful things created by those with broken hearts who do not give up but rather find amazing ways to reach out and help others. Although you may not be there yet, you may be later. Just keep the door open and your heart warmed to this possibility.

However, if it is still early, please know that it is completely normal for you to be sad, to feel alone in your grief, and to wonder if you'll survive it. You will feel emotionally drained at times. You'll need to do things to reenergize, or as we sometimes say, to "refill your well that has gone dry." You will find the first holidays and anniversaries especially difficult and deep feelings may resurface during such times, despite your best efforts to control them. We are here to tell you that you will survive it with hard work and with the support of others. Support services and details are listed in the resources at the end of this book, and we encourage you to seek support. One mom shares this simple but critical message: "Take your time to grieve, because your loved baby has died. Be an active participant in your healing."

POSTTRAUMATIC GROWTH

A poor prenatal diagnosis has long-term consequences, both socially and psychologically, for the parents who experience it. While writing this book, Stephanie conducted research on the impact of receiving a prenatal diagnosis (Azri, 2014). Many women we have spoken with developed posttraumatic growth symptoms following the loss, as did we. They became involved in supporting other women, creating helpful Facebook pages, mentoring others, writing books, and developing personally or within their relationships. It may take months or years before you are ready to see the positives, the growth. However, this is an amazing legacy for our children. Although it does not take away the pain, it can bring a measure of peace in our hearts knowing that our little ones made a difference, no matter how short their lives. At present, you may not believe that your loss could bring forth anything positive but watch and be ready for your own posttraumatic growth.

GRIEF RESOURCES OFFER GUIDANCE

There are countless books that describe grief and mourning, and there are online resources, community resources, counseling, and other options available. Believe you can make it. Embrace the need to grieve and jump in.

Pastor and grief expert Doug Manning writes in his book, *Don't Take My Grief Away*, "Grief is not an enemy, it is a friend. It is the natural process of walking through the hurt and growing through the walk. Stand up tall to your friends and say, Don't take my grieve away from me. I deserve it and I'm going to have it." Will you allow yourself to feel it?

TIPS AND ADVICE

* Remember that grief is a journey. It doesn't start and stop at any given time. It continues throughout life and although it is a normal part of life, it is often excruciatingly painful.

- Acknowledge the roller coaster of emotions that you are feeling. Expect the bad days and respect and appreciate the good days. Accept either without fighting it. You will go through it and come out on the other side. But it will take much work over time. Understand that from now on things will be different; you will be different. But different doesn't mean that everything will be bad and hard, either.

- Allow yourself to feel. Many try to distract themselves from their pain. However, your grief will catch up with you eventually. Feeling grief is acknowledging love, and it is a healthy process.

- Seek support. Although grief is healthy and necessary, it is still very painful and overwhelming. Talk to someone. Seek out one of the many infant loss experts who will be able to assist you and help you to deal with your natural, raw emotions.

- Find others who have experienced similar losses and have gained some health during the grief journey. Whether online, face to face, or on the phone, share your thoughts and feelings with others who also "get it." Stephanie kept an online journal since finding out that her daughter Talina would die, which shows the evolution in her grief journey over a decade. We hope you will feel the growth and hope as well as the realism of life after loss. You may read it at www.PDSAustralia.org/journalsteph.html.

- Be attentive about how your grief is developing. Although grief is normal, some women develop postnatal depression or anxiety following a poor prenatal diagnosis or the death of a baby. If you are not able to cope or if you have thoughts of hurting yourself or others, seek professional help immediately.

- Although you may feel powerless and out of control, know that you are not alone in this. How you move through this process of loving and letting go is yours to create and to own. There are others who do understand and might be there for you. As you will see someday, when you give to others, gifts come back to you. If you allow others to help you, you also help them to feel grateful and appreciated. They are parenting their child as they give to you. Your turn will come and then you will understand. In the meantime, give this grief journey all you have. Your love was—and is—that deep. No one who dies should be forgotten too soon. With this loss comes the opportunity to change and grow, to mature and learn, and eventually to feel gratefulness that your child lived and was loved by you.

24

DOWN THE ROAD A BIT

NO ROAD MAP

If you have made it through the first weeks and months after your child died, you might think it should be smoother sailing ahead. It is common to feel like you shouldn't cry as much, be as angry, or think about the loss of your baby as much. But you do and you are.

The road to recovery is long after losing a precious little one. You may feel lost and out of control at times, yet you may feel calm and some peace at others. You can't predict what will happen when, so find a way to go with the flow even if you are not that kind of a person. Healing and grief do not come in prescribed stages and phases. You may have many feelings but not in a specific order, and sometimes you have a lot of feelings all at once. You may need to retreat. The grief experience rarely can be controlled and there is no road map. Feelings can come and go for no apparent reason. There are some days where they peak and are more intense. Strong emotions may surface when watching a commercial, when in the baby aisle at the grocery store, when invited to baptisms and baby showers, and when you hear certain music or experience certain smells. Expect this to happen when you least expect it. Bring tissue with you everywhere, be prepared to excuse yourself when necessary, and know that this is how it goes now in your life, at least for a while.

Some people say that they lost the first six (or many more) months of their life. They don't remember all that happened, what they did, who came to visit, or much else. Parents (and all those who are grieving) often say that they also become forgetful. You may find the iron in the refrigerator, the television remote on the phone cradle, and many items misplaced or lost. Although this is frustrating, appreciate the humor in it. Keep lists (taped to the cupboard or on the refrigerator) to help you cope and function. Asking others for grace and forgiveness up front might be a good idea, and give *yourself* grace and understanding. You are amid a swirling sea, barely keeping your head above water.

FIND SUPPORT

Make sure that you have support. People who can finish your sentences for you. People who take care of and pamper you. People who bolster your self-confidence and love you no matter what. People who help you find joy and beauty in the world, even when you don't see it. Whether in-person support or social media, find it and use it as often as it feels right. And if you find that people are saying things that are not supportive, either remove yourself from their presence (or unfriend them on Facebook) or tell them what you need and what is not helpful. If they cannot provide it to you, it may be because they are incapable of that now. You might find it helpful to tell them that you need other things from people right now so as not to increase your pain. Therefore, you are taking a break and hope that they understand. Whether they do or not, don't let drama or pressure add to your burden. Taking care of yourself and finding support is important.

Of course, things will go wrong and you will feel overwhelmed with uncontrollable emotions. This is what happens when we love deeply and our loved one is absent from our everyday lives. Some days you feel like a basket case. Or you find ways to "look the part" of the person you used to be while you crumble inside. Be honest with yourself, your partner, and others during this time, which lasts a while but not forever.

SPECIAL DAYS AND HOLIDAYS

Some of the difficult days you will face are the "firsts": the due date, birth and death anniversaries, and holidays, especially Mother's and

Father's days and Christmas/Passover. Although in the beginning, it is the weekly and then monthly anniversaries that are significant. There are resources to help you prepare for and handle these important days. *Coping with the Holidays and Celebrations* (Ilse) is one that is easy to read and offers specific suggestions for things you can do to help you cope.

Prior to these special days, consider what you want to do and make plans. How will you spend the day, and if you celebrate or gather, who do you want to be there? What special things will you do? Some people realize that having a plan gives them more control rather than letting things happen, which can sometimes lead to disappointment if others don't provide you what you need (a Mother's Day card, a gift for the Christmas tree, an acknowledgement about the specialness of the day, a moment when your child is remembered).

Reminding people can be helpful. It might be better if you tell them in person or on the phone. Probably there are not many mind readers in your family and community. Ask yourself, "How will others know what will help me and what I want, unless I tell them?" To be clear, people can be clueless about what to say and how to help. Often they cannot even guess what will be helpful; thus, they easily make mistakes and everyone feels even worse. Without guidance from you, they will make lots of mistakes. Then there are those who cannot come through, even when you tell them what would be helpful. Probably if you look at their personality, you will recognize that they don't cope well or aren't good at honoring the needs of others. They likely never were, and they won't be good at it now, either. When a whole family is drowning in the ocean, is that the time to teach (or to expect) someone to learn a new stroke? This loss affects everyone in some way.

> I bought Hannah a Mother's Day card from the twins (who died). Then I went back and forth and back and forth with this thought: "Throw it in the garbage?" "Give it to her?" "Garbage?" "Give it to her?" Finally, I gave it to her and she was very grateful. I just didn't know what was the right thing to do. How do you know? —John

WHAT HAPPENS WHEN SOME OF THE SHOCK WEARS OFF?

Sometimes after around four to six months after a loss, parents say that things seem worse. Almost as if they were underwater, which kept them numb. Now things are beginning to become clear and more evident. The feelings of missing your baby do not go away but may intensify. Why would this happen, you may wonder. Shouldn't things be getting better?

> I remember crying every single day for six months. Toward the end of that time I remember feeling horrible. It seemed that the pain was even more sharp and hard to deal with than when our baby first died. Later I realized that it is a common occurrence and did not last long. And now I understand why. —A mom

Around this time, the meals have stopped coming, the mailbox is empty, shock begins to lift, the nightmare hasn't ended, and the reality that this is real and forever is combined with feeling very alone. The world has continued for others, while your clock has stopped and you are still stuck amid the tragedy, the time warp. This can be a scary time and you may wonder if it will always be like this. Thankfully, it does change and can improve. You just have to understand what is going on, work to accept this stage as temporary, know it is common and a normal part of the healing process, and then move on.

One way to look at this is to imagine a river with both peaceful, calm spots and roaring rapids over sharp rocks with lots of twists and turns. If you can allow yourself to be in that river and not fight it (or feel guilty) about those calm and maybe even happy moments, do it. Then there will be days when you are stuck in the churning, icy waters waiting to be sucked under. Don't fight these times, either. Let yourself be amid the pain. Accept it as a reminder of the depth of your love for your baby, the price we pay for love. It won't last forever, we are sure of that, so let the water flow over you and "go big"—give in to your grief for a short while knowing that calm is ahead and some peace will come.

Some therapists suggest that you make appointments with your grief. Pick a time and limit the length—maybe Thursdays from 7 until 8:30 pm. Then ready yourself and the room with mementos, candles, music, and whatever thoughts come forth. Be with your loved one and allow the natural feelings of mourning flow. At the end of your "appointment," do something to transition—meditate, pray, say a few words out loud to your baby or yourself—then shut it down, put things away, and do something else. You can always make more appointments. You will find that the grief does not just go away, but it may not need to be continually present, either.

FAMILY AND FRIENDS

As time goes on, fewer people will remember that you are still grieving. They may not remember you on the holidays; they may say things that give you the impression that they think you should move on. Unless they have had a significant loss and really do understand, it is likely that their support and sensitivity to your pain and continuing mourning will lessen over time. This is not done to purposely hurt you. They have moved on. Their life goes on in a normal way. Although they may think of you often and want to reach out, they may worry that they will hurt you more by reminding you of your loss. If you think about it, you might have done this, too. A relative or a friend may have had a loved one—or even their beloved pet—die and they hurt for a long time. Yet, if you are like most of us, you may have been there for them in the beginning, but didn't you go on with your life soon after? And when you thought of them, did you give a call, send a card or flowers, go out for a meal, or invite them over months later? Most of us can't sustain that long-term support. However, hopefully you have a friend or relative (or two) who do get it and hang in with you for the long haul. Or maybe you have met some people at the local support group or online who are there for you. Possibly there is someone in your faith community who brings you light and love on a regular basis. If you don't have this but need it, you'll probably have to seek it out. There are plenty of ways to find support in the resources at the back of this book.

> I remember wanting to shout from the rooftops: my baby has died. The world needs to *stop*. How can you all go about your business like nothing happened? My world has ended. —Anonymous

If you feel let down or need more from others, tell them. You could write them a note or e-mail gently encouraging them to be there for you. Tell them what helps (talking and them listening or getting out of the house for some fun) and see if they will support you in that way. A special request for help can be a relief to others. It makes it easier for them to give because they know just what you need. In this case, both parties usually win. They want to help but don't know how, and you need help so you tell them what you need. Don't be shy unless you want to stay that way.

WHAT NEXT?

Whether it is time to consider another baby (if that is an option) or you need more time to heal, such decisions are weighty ones. Many parents talk about being on different wavelengths or timelines than their partners. So if this is the case for you, know that you are not alone.

Another baby cannot fix this. Ask any parent who had a subsequent child after a loss and you will learn that getting pregnant was often complicated, the pregnancy was the world's longest, and if the baby lived (most do, but to be honest, lightning can strike twice) the parents were changed. Love for the new baby can be slow to develop and fears can be overwhelming at times. When you are ready for a new baby (or if you become pregnant before you felt you were ready), take it one day at a time and avoid projecting or adding to your basket of fear if you can help it. This baby will never replace the earlier baby, any more than a new husband can replace the previous one. Instead, see this as a new chapter and realize that this baby is a new baby who deserves your love for who he is. You will find many positives with your pregnancy, and when you realize that your baby is alive and healthy, you will celebrate and find happiness again. You may find it helpful to read more about subsequent pregnancies and rainbow babies in chapters 25 and 26.

If you are not able to have another child or need time to decide, go with that. Seek other joys in your life (pets, nieces and nephews, gardening, supporting others who have had tragedies, taking on new work challenges, baking, etc.), not that these other activities can fix anything—they can't. But you can only be down and out for so long before it gets complicated, difficult, and old. You can still be the loving parent to your child who has died. You can still honor, remember, and include your baby in your heart on a daily basis. You will know when you are ready—or your partner may suggest that it is time—to do things that bring you light and make you feel proud and happy. Just as you might have made an appointment with your grief, make an appointment with some activity that brings you joy.

Remember that you are still the parent to your child who has died. Forever. So don't feel that you have to forget or that you can't say his name out loud. Rather, seek your own special ways to be inclusive and to share your child with others. You may even find some mission or creative venture that honors and helps you—and others—to remember him. In time, you will find that thoughts of your baby no longer consume your every waking moment anymore.

> After awhile I realized that I could live again, have some fun, be creative, think of another baby, and not feel guilty. My daughter has a special place inside me and in our family. I don't have to worry she will be forgotten, because she won't. This frees me up to live my life. There are certain moments or days when I feel blue or miss her so terribly. But it is no longer every day and that is good. —A mom

INTIMACY

Having intimate relationships with a partner can be difficult for some women who associate sex with procreation. If this is the case for you, you may find it difficult to enjoy intimacy without the memories of the baby that passed away flashing in your mind or without accepting the fact that sex may not lead to a pregnancy. Try to remember sex before having children. Try to remember the time when you and your partner simply enjoyed intimacy, with no other emotional burdens, and how important this was for your relationship. Take it slowly. You may decide to be intimate without sex. For example, practice hugs, hand holding, and romantic gestures, so that when the time comes, sex is an extension of your love rather than a reminder of what you've lost.

TIPS AND ADVICE

- Be patient. Allow yourself to rediscover you, your partner, and the rest of your life. It may take time to feel comfortable being intimate or to discuss children. Talk about your thoughts and your fears and start slowly (hold hands, talk about nonthreatening subjects, etc.).

- Be prepared for things to get worse before they get better. A lot of people tend to think that after the funeral, things will start getting better. The truth is often the opposite, though this is not always the case. After the funeral, friends and relatives might move on with their lives, your employer may ask when you're coming back, partners may return to work, and you may have to face daily life on your own. Things generally get tough between four and six months after the death of a baby and are very difficult periodically until after the first anniversary. After the first year, things slowly get better for most people, but the truth is that things may be difficult for a while. If you experience this, do not be alarmed. Many moms do get worse before they get better, but eventually they get there, too.

- When you're ready to resume your "normal" life, start slowly. You may decide to go grocery shopping for a few things or simply to make a few phone calls. Do not try to take too much on at once; gradually take on more.

- Be mindful that no matter how much time has passed, there will be special events that will trigger your grief. Accept that there will always be bad days (for example, anniversaries, holidays, etc.).

- Forgive others around you. As time goes on, friends and relatives assume that you have moved on and stop remembering dates or events. This can be painful to you, but unfortunately it happens to most people. Although it is painful, forgive those who do not know your pain.

- Accept that your life is different. Life has changed forever. You are no longer innocent. You will no longer believe that life will always be safe for you. And as you learn to deal with this knowledge, you will need to learn to navigate this new truth and find peace and eventual happiness within it.

25

TRYING AGAIN

As you contemplate another pregnancy, you will find you have mixed emotions. This is a big step and if this is an option, you will want to prepare yourself for the journey of trying again.

NEVER FORGETTING

Your precious baby is irreplaceable. Another cannot fill your baby's place. Know for sure that your child will always be within your heart, holding her own space. Also know that you can continue to love the baby who lives with challenges and yet want another. Now take a breath. Yes, breathe. And when ready—if ready—open your heart to prepare yourself for another child, knowing that this baby will be his own person. This is a risky but loving, courageous step to take. Of course, there are no guarantees about whether you can get pregnant again or how it will work out.

Considering another pregnancy or finding out that you are expecting another baby should be one of the most exciting times in your life. However, your experience is different. Your expectations are no longer naive. Fear comes easily to those who have had a bad outcome. You may wonder if it could happen again or if you could cope with another loss if it comes to that. Understandably, you might wonder if you have enough love for another baby, knowing you can't replace her.

CONCERNS

Your concerns are many. For some, it is fear—the feeling that a poor prenatal diagnosis could strike again or even that a miscarriage or still-birth could happen. You may fear that you won't know how to cope if something terrible happens. For others, it is loyalty—the feeling that you are disrespecting the memory of your baby by having another one or replacing your child who lives with challenges. Perhaps you fear that you may not have enough love for another baby. Whatever your fears, deciding to move forward with a new pregnancy is a complex step. This is indeed an emotionally charged time. Sometimes partners can't agree on the timing, or they feel anxious discussing a new baby at all.

WHAT IF YOU ARE UNABLE TO GET PREGNANT AGAIN?

It might be that there will be no subsequent baby for you. Maybe due to age, infertility problems, or even the potential risks of another pregnancy, you won't have another. You may decide that your family is complete and accept that as well as you can, even if it is not your choice. Or maybe your relationship has not bounced back after the loss; disagreements and tension may get in the way. Perhaps you struggle with the reality that you can't get pregnant or can't afford to pay the costs for more medical procedures or adoption. Maybe your partner does not want to try again or adopt. It could be that you both want another baby but that the pregnancy and all the problems you have had make it too scary. This is especially true if mom's health was the reason the pregnancy ended prematurely or if the recurrence rate is high for another baby with similar problems. Many partners suggest that they are unwilling to take the risk that that could happen again. Other parents go to great lengths to avoid ending childbearing with a traumatic loss.

When couples simply cannot agree about whether to try for another baby, it can cause tension. The same is true of infertility issues. Conflicts may revolve about health, social, financial, or emotional reasons, such as the fear that there may be no more babies. None of this changes the fact that you may have to grieve the loss of all future babies as well as the one who died. This can be confusing for parents. Although you may feel this way now, give it time and talk. You never know what can happen—in fact, sometimes a spontaneous pregnancy occurs, which can be a welcome surprise.

It may also be that as a couple you are having trouble getting along right now, struggling through your altered life since the loss of your baby or parenting your child who lives. The tension is understandable, yet it can be destructive if you are not careful. Perhaps by making your relationship a priority and working through your grief, you can reclaim your loving and warm partnership. How you are getting along as a couple may influence your decisions about trying again. At present, there are only a few books written to help couples cope, communicate, and better understand each other. You can find them listed in the resources at the end of this book.

If you are single and the father has disappeared or is unreliable, your struggles for another baby are complicated about how and if to get pregnant again. You may want to think this through. Do you want to wait until you find a steady partner or do you want to seek assisted reproduction options? Maybe you want to look into adoption, which can be difficult without a partner. It is also possible that you want to give yourself some time to see how things develop. In any case, you will need support, so look for nonjudgmental friends or family members who will listen and be there for you.

Whatever your situation, you now have some struggles, some feelings, and some decisions ahead. Many women seem to have a hard time accepting the end of childbearing. There may be a mental tug-of-war about what to do. You may find yourself searching for a variety of solutions. For example, you may consider medical alternatives like in vitro fertilization, surrogacy, donors, or other options like adoption, foster care, or other opportunities to have another baby in your life.

> After our baby died thirty-five years ago, we trained to become foster parents of babies and have been doing that ever since. It was our way of having babies in our home and giving back. We are grateful we had this opportunity; it helped us find happiness again. —Parents of Mary

DETERMINING WHEN YOU ARE READY

Some parents know immediately that they want to try again. Others say they'll never try again. Perspectives can change with time and different circumstances. Some say the thought of another pregnancy cripples them with fear, and others are so anxious that it is almost unbearable. This is a complicated time when hope is mixed with fear.

> I remember leaving the day of the funeral telling myself that I would not ever replace her, that having babies would end with her. And then, some months later, this gut-wrenching need to hold a baby overtook me. It was almost primal; there were no discussions about it. It would happen and my husband knew it. —Stephanie

It is common for moms to describe an irrational gut feeling, rather than a well-thought-out plan, that indicates the time is right to try again. Some moms simply *know* when the time is right. They wake up one morning knowing that they are ready. No one else can tell you when the timing is right for you. A warm feeling of contentment may come over you when you are ready. You will probably be afraid and anxious, but despite this, you will be willing to take the chance and try for another baby. You might suddenly find yourself pregnant before you even thought it through. If this happens, you cannot go back. Stay positive and recognize that you may need to put your present grief on hold in order to get through the pregnancy, which is hard. Another option is to work harder at your mourning with help from a counselor or others who understand as you seek ways to continue to parent the baby who died while also feeling joy and hope about the baby on the way.

Your situation might be complicated by concern that you could receive another poor prognosis. The baby's problem could be genetic or there might be high rate of recurrence. You may need to visit with your provider to learn about your options. No matter your situation, if you are pregnant again, you will need reassurance and support to keep your anxiety and worries in check. Since your baby may pick up on such emotions, being as physically and emotionally healthy as you can prior to and during the pregnancy will be important.

Are You Physically Ready?

Visit your midwife, obstetrician, or family doctor to ensure good health prior to becoming pregnant. Many doctors recommend a minimum of six months before trying to conceive again. This depends, of course, on your personal circumstances, the gestational age at the time of the birth, the type of birth (vaginal versus caesarean versus dilation and curettage), and how well you recovered. If possible, you may want to consider timing another pregnancy to avoid being on the same cycle as your last loss. It can be challenging to have a similar due date with clinic visits on the previous schedule. This makes it harder—though not impossible—to keep the babies and births separate.

During pregnancy, your body uses vitamins and minerals to aid the growing baby, so be sure to replenish your body with healthy eating, exercise, and vitamins and minerals before becoming pregnant, if you can.

Are You Emotionally Ready?

It's somewhat easier to know if you are physically ready than it is to know whether you are emotionally ready to conceive again. It is much more difficult to assess. No one but you can decide if you are emotionally ready, though you can seek advice and feedback from your therapist or support group leader, who may be able to offer you ideas regarding what questions to ask yourself. Discussing this with your partner early on and throughout is, of course, important.

Talk to other bereaved mothers, friends, family, or a counselor. Grieving your loss well and allowing yourself to heal while parenting a special needs child are important before considering another baby. Some questions we suggest that you ask yourself include: Have I grieved well? Do I cry every day for my baby? Is there some happiness and hope in my life? Do I want another baby to fill my empty arms or am I ready to seek another distinct and special little life? Do I have the love and energy it takes to parent this special needs child and to have another? What if it happens again—how will I cope? Am I getting the help I need to do healthy grief work from others who have been there or from a support group, counselor, or clergy? Do I feel I am ready to give myself to a new baby? Could I cope if I received another poor prenatal diagnosis? How will I deal with this stress? Who could I turn to for support?

Considering such questions before making a decision can be helpful for you and your partner. No matter how much you want to fill your arms, a new baby will not replace the one who died, and there are no guarantees that the next child will be healthy. Understanding that can help you to prepare and bond with a new baby in a healthy manner.

Although many family members are supportive, you may need to brace yourself for some "concerns." Others may feel that you are not ready. Hear this message, even if you don't want to. What are their reasons? They could be afraid for you or see issues with your emotional health and are trying to warn you. On the other hand, they may wonder why you would risk more potential pain. Some may suggest adoption while others might suggest that you should be satisfied with the children you already have. Other comments may be unhelpful to you. Even if meant to be supportive, such comments can be hurtful. Try to consider their positions without judging them too harshly. Evaluate whether you think their concerns hold any merit or if they are being protective of you.

> When an acquaintance found out I was pregnant again, she glared at me and my stomach and said, "What do you want? To be the one who dies next time?" She obviously wanted me to know that she disapproved. —Stephanie

EMOTIONS WHILE TRYING TO BECOME PREGNANT

If you feel desperate for a baby or are scared that something could happen again, your emotions will run high. It may be difficult to enjoy the pregnancy, but you cheat both yourself and your baby if you don't, so work on those emotions beforehand. Take some time, talk with others, bring it up with your support group, and tell yourself not to rush into something if it feels frantic and hurried. You are probably not quite ready.

Don't be surprised if you have feelings of guilt. It is common to wonder how you dare replace your loved baby who died or who has serious problems. You may even wonder if you are a horrible parent, if you have enough love left for another child, or if you can ever love another child as much as you love the baby who died or who is ill. Even mothers who had healthy babies admit that this is a concern sometimes. You may recognize that the attention that will go to another child will impact the time you have to care for your special needs baby or to grieve for the baby who died. This is something to consider when contemplating your readiness for another baby. These feelings of guilt and confusion may come when you least expect them. Knowing that this is normal may help.

The truth is, guilt is a common and strong emotion for someone who is grieving. For many, feeling pain is better than not feeling anything at all, so you may have a need to hold on to your grief as your connection to your child who has died or who lives with issues. However, you don't have to hold on to the guilt or sad feelings to be connected with your child. As Lori's group leader asked her, "What could you do with your energy and your life if you let go of the deep sadness and used your feelings of love for good?" That question was a game changer for Lori. She realized she could still hold on to her son and keep her love intact without focusing on only the grief and sadness. From that point on, she shifted her mind-set to be as positive as possible and to become productive by helping others.

Share any emotional burden you carry as you consider another pregnancy. Seek advice and support during this process from professionals and those who have been there.

MANAGING YOUR ANXIETY AFTER BECOMING PREGNANT

Becoming pregnant again is only the beginning of the roller coaster ride. Some women become anxious once pregnant, and others go to their calm, hopeful place. You can drive yourself crazy imagining all the things that could go wrong. Instead, work on enjoying your pregnancy. What if this was all the time you get with this baby? Would you want it to be full of stress and worry? While you certainly hope and pray that your baby will be healthy this time, do what you can to think positively and send happy, hopeful, and positive energy to your baby, to yourself, and to your partner. You deserve some happiness and hope. Work to bring that to this pregnancy as much as you can.

Once you've become pregnant and announced it, it's time to put a stress management plan in place for the remainder of the pregnancy. The first step is to surround yourself with support. As stated above, seek friends, family, and support groups that deal with subsequent pregnancies.

While trying to be positive and hopeful, it is okay to speak about your fears, thoughts, and feelings. Get them out of your head and heart. Share them aloud if that helps. If you don't have anyone to speak them to, write the thoughts in a journal or a letter to your angel or living child or to your growing baby. Or find a subsequent pregnancy social media group. You may choose to keep what you've written or to burn it afterward.

Remember that most everything you are feeling is normal, from overbearing love to overbearing guilt. Work on your attachment to your new baby.

Be prepared to erect your protective shield when it comes to reactions from others once you are pregnant. Many friends and strangers ask mothers-to-be about pregnancy. Some of the questions asked may include: How many children do you have? What number is this for you? Are you excited about this baby? Most comments are genuinely caring but nevertheless can make you feel anxious. You may find it helpful to have a few planned responses for various people and situations. For example, you could say, "We have had a previous loss. This pregnancy is precious and precarious. Thank you for asking." Another option is, "I appreciate your concern. I'd prefer not to talk about it here."

THE SAME OR DIFFERENT MEDICAL FACILITIES?

Returning to the same hospital, clinic, or office during your pregnancy may trigger bittersweet emotions. During the pregnancy and after the birth, you may find that your feelings flow between sadness and hopefulness, as you remember your earlier pregnancy. However, you may wish to limit those reminders during the birth and postnatal checkups by requesting a different room. Some mothers work through their grief and get to the point where they feel that they can better overcome such feelings by being in the same room. Think that one through and decide what works best for you.

I was not ready for the myriad of emotions I felt the first time I walked past the delivery room [where] I birthed my daughter the year before. I was so happy going in this time to have a healthy baby, but I still felt confused. —Anna

On Brennan's one-year anniversary, I visited the hospital where he was born. I was expecting another baby soon and needed to make some peace with the place that brought such heartache before I returned to have another baby. While clearly upset and anxious, I did a few very special things that helped. I cried, relived every moment I could remember, and wrote Brennan a poem. Then I visited with my midwife about the past and about the next time I would be in the labor and delivery wing delivering another baby. Shortly afterward, surprisingly, I took a little nap. Such peace and calm I felt after an emotional few hours. I felt renewed hope for a healthy baby. — Sherokee

You may also have the option of changing hospitals or clinics. If that feels better and you can do so, you should. In either case, make sure that the staff know about your loss so that they can be sensitive and make appropriate plans. Tell them what would be helpful (this is where a birth plan can be helpful). It is important too that you allow yourself to feel this joy freely and to remain in the present during the birth of your new baby. Enjoy this beautiful time.

ONE DAY AT A TIME

Finally, remember to take one day at a time. Don't think ahead to the birth if that is a traumatic thought; just enjoy each day as it comes. Don't dwell on the tests that you fear; enjoy each little kick, every scan, and every moment that your baby is sweetly snuggled inside of you. You will never replace your angel baby or give up on your child with special needs, but you will learn that you have the capacity to love another child just as much. A subsequent pregnancy can be a challenging journey, but once you hold your baby at your breast, it will be worth it.

We both agreed that seven years of trying and multiple miscarriages was wearing us down. Being over forty, we really didn't think there was much chance of [conceiving and] continuing to torture ourselves. What a shock it was then to discover I was pregnant at forty-one! Each scan we had was obviously terrifying. When our son, Ciaran, was finally born, I found that all my previous pregnancy losses became insignificant compared to the joy I felt having a "rainbow baby." It was as if a darkness that had hung over us had lifted and we embarked on our new journey—parenthood. —Bernie

Before you start trying for another baby, consider the following tips and advice.

TIPS AND ADVICE

- Do not rush into this decision. Take your time to decide whether you're ready or not. Ask yourself about your reasons for wanting—or not wanting—another baby.
- Ensure that you've grieved for your baby. Make sure that you've taken the time to say good-bye properly and that you are ready to have a new baby—not trying to replace the baby who has died.
- Consider how you would feel if you had the same gender as the baby who died? Would it matter? What if there was something wrong with this new pregnancy? Would you be able to do it again?
- Seek medical advice. Are you medically cleared for another pregnancy? What are the medical or genetic implications of trying again?
- Talk to your partner. How does he feel about it? What are your thoughts as a couple? Have you taken the time to really discuss it and hear one another's point of view?
- If single, talk it through with others whom you trust. Discuss how you will cope and live with a baby and no partner. Secure the support you can ahead of time; you will need it.
- Join a support group and ask others about their experiences, joys, and trials. Share your own emotional struggles, fears, and hopes.
- If you become pregnant, you will need to come to grips with your feelings, fears, and hopes. Which will override the others? Will you let fear and worry prevail, stealing your joy and hope? Or will you nurture this baby to the fullest, sending messages of love and the belief that all will be well? Since babies can hear your voice during pregnancy, can they also sense your feelings? What message do you want him to feel? You could not control your previous pregnancy—

nor this one—but you can make choices about your attitude and about the way you show your love and the way you deal with your fears. As a pregnancy-after-loss Facebook support group asks, "Will you choose hope over fear while nurturing your grief?" No one can decide that for you. It is up to you. There are books to help you during this time, two of which are *Another Baby? Maybe*, by Shero-kee Ilse and Maribeth Doerr, and *When Pregnancy Follows Loss*, by Joann O'Leary.

> Seeing pregnant women was a whole world of pain—and naturally they seemed to be everywhere. Why could they do it, but I couldn't? Every moment of every day was tarnished by the fact that we had lost our baby. In January, my husband and I agreed to try again for a baby. I made it very clear that if things went wrong this time, I would not be attempting a third time. —Mandy

- Only time will tell if you have another baby. Life is unpredictable. This is a journey that requires trust, faith, hope, and lots of courage. Believe that you will cope and live through whatever happens.

26

SUBSEQUENT BABIES

If you are fortunate, you will have an easy pregnancy and bring a healthy baby home. We hope so. This is a new beginning for you, and yet it is a continuation of the story. Your child who came before will be in your heart as you hold this new baby; they are intertwined, which means that this birth is not all roses for most parents. Yet you will find gratitude that your empty arms are no longer empty. And if you are still parenting your child who preceded this little one, you will find ways to care for and love both.

It is possible that you may not have had a healthy rainbow baby, since on rare occasions, problems can occur again. In that unlikely scenario, use the resources and support you have previously found to live through this next experience. Amazingly, you survived it once; you can do it again if necessary. If your baby is not healthy, you may feel that you are spinning out of control. This was not your plan, though it may have been your fear. You now may be revisiting those feelings of helplessness and experiencing disbelief, medical discussions that hurt your head and heart, flashbacks, and more. Like most people, you feel you deserved a happy ending. Why should you have to experience loss? Anything less than a healthy baby can be felt as another loss. Once again, you may wonder how you will make it. You can make it with help and guidance from others. Ask for it, pray for it, seek it out. Some of the previous chapters may be helpful.

CELEBRATION AND REMINDERS: FEELING HAPPY AND SAD

If your baby is healthy, it will be time to celebrate. The depth of your feelings may surprise you. Such relief! You will be amazed at what it feels like to have a healthy, living baby after all that you have been through. Having a subsequent healthy baby is an answer to hope and prayer. You may be so excited to have your baby in your home. You have waited so long for this and worried so much that there would be problems. Feelings of euphoria may continue for a long time, along with gratefulness that you both survived and now have hope for the future.

You and others in your family may think that your sad and painful emotions will disappear with a healthy baby in your arms; however, it rarely works like that. Your new baby may be a reminder of what you missed last time. Feelings of grief, sorrow, or even numbness can occur when you least expect it. One baby does not replace another. Indeed, you may realize that this subsequent birth is bittersweet. Bonding issues have been known to occur, especially during the first hours and days. However, knowing you can have feelings of both sadness and happiness, as well as grief and hope, allows the love for your baby to shine through.

There will be times when you think of your previous baby and realize how much you miss her. Many mothers and fathers have shared that they were stunned by the pull on their hearts. It may help to know that this commonly happens and that you have the right—because you love them both—to hurt inside for all that could have been. Someday, you may come to realize—as many of us have—that without the short life of the baby who died, this new child might not be here at all. It is an awesome and amazing thought. If you are not ready for it now, put it away for later or let it go if need be. If your child still lives, this healthy baby will be a reminder of what could have been and what you are missing. This is also bittersweet.

Many parents find the joy slow to come. In the 2014 film *Return to Zero*, based on a true story, Maggie, the mother of a rainbow baby, asks the doctor after her healthy daughter's birth, "When does the joy come?" Even after a healthy birth come vivid reminders of the previous child. Oh, what could have been! Those months fearing that it could happen again could have served as a road block to your complete bonding and love. Having this baby does not mean that you will experience instant joy and that life is perfect again. In fact, that naïveté that you lost never quite comes back. You may always carry some sense of vulnerability. The joy comes, but might take its time as this baby wraps herself around and through your heart.

It is common for moms and dads to worry about "moving on" after having another baby. You may feel like you have forgotten or abandoned your previous child. Or, if she's still alive, you may feel as if you don't tend her as much as you did before this baby. You may wonder if you should feel this happy. Again, you are not alone. This is commonly reported by parents, but it does not last long for most. In fact, there are a number of support groups for parents with subsequent pregnancies. A Facebook group called PALS (Pregnancy after Loss Support) offers a closed community of parents who help each other during and after the birth of rainbow babies.

You may even think that you do not deserve to be happy again, particularly if you chose to terminate your pregnancy after a poor prenatal diagnosis, but you do have the right to feel happy and full of hope again. Embrace it and go with it. No one should give you the impression that past decisions or circumstances need to interfere with your beloved baby and this jubilant time in your life. Go forth with gusto and know that you can always nurture your feelings for your angel baby while still loving her sibling in your arms and in your home.

Remember that you can never replace a baby. Remember that your baby who died loves you. She would not want you to be sad for the rest of your life. And the truth is, it is physically impossible to be sad and cry for the rest of your life. Eventually, you have to heal; you deserve to feel joy as you dare to love again. You baby would want it that way.

> I found myself in a shopping center with my mom looking at Christmas ornaments. While I was looking for a "baby's first Christmas" ornament for my newborn son, my mom came over to me with a nice little angel and told me that would be great to go on my daughter's grave. I looked at her and said, "I don't want to think about it. I don't want to be sad. My baby's going to be here for Christmas and I want to be happy." I had just done what I swore I wouldn't ever do, what I tried so hard to imagine. I had consciously decided to put her death aside and to focus on his life. The loss of guilt was liberating.
> —Stephanie

Hold within yourself positive and uplifting thoughts. Surround yourself with hopeful people and seek parents who have undertaken subsequent pregnancies. It is important to be able to learn from others who survived and who dealt with the mixed feelings that come with a subsequent baby.

IMPACT OF GENDER

Some parents experience mixed emotions with the birth of a child of a specific gender. Some prefer to have a baby of the opposite gender so as to reserve a special place in their hearts for the baby who died, while others prefer a baby of the same gender so as to get another chance to do things the way they were hoping. This may be also true if your baby with challenges still lives. You will be comparing the two and might have preferred one gender over another. Perhaps even sharing the clothes and toys is easier and more special when the children are the same gender. Each person has his or her own hopes and expectations. Not everyone will understand the significance of the baby's gender. After all, you should be grateful to have a healthy baby—and of course you are—but gender issues may complicate your emotions.

> I never wanted to replace Talina. But I was desperate to give Julianna another sister to play with. Watching my young daughter ask whether she could please have a sister every time I became pregnant broke my heart and to birth four sons in a row made Talina's loss much more real for her and me. —Stephanie

You may need time to adjust and get used to your baby's gender. This is normal and nothing to be ashamed of. You probably know in your heart that your baby is precious, no matter what gender. Don't let this issue complicate your love and your future with this much-anticipated child. Hopefully, soon after birth you are able to work through this issue and love this child for who she is. As she becomes a person in her own unique right, her gender will have less of an impact over time. If gender becomes a hurdle you just can't get over, counseling is a good idea. You don't want to hold resentment over time and you don't want your child scarred for life because she feels unwanted. Of course, you may not have an issue with gender and feel only thankfulness and gratitude.

IMPACT OF AGE DIFFERENCE

The death of a baby—or the need to adjust to the care considerations of your child with challenges—may create a bigger age gap than you preferred or anticipated. Your living children—and even adults around you—may express some disappointment about the age gap, which may trigger feelings in you.

> There was now four years between my eldest and youngest son. This should have been a two-year gap. The hardest was to know that the age gap was too big. They would never play together and people made sure to remind me. —Helen

It is important to remind yourself that you are not responsible for the gap between children. This is not something you can change. The significance of age gaps decreases with time; a four-year age gap may seem large when children are young, but as they mature, age gaps become less obvious or relevant. People who comment about the age gap may not know the reasons for it or may not realize the impact of what they're saying. Give them grace, if you can.

HOW MANY CHILDREN DO YOU HAVE?

If your baby died, one of the hardest questions that you, as a bereaved mom, can be asked is how many children you have. It is excruciating, especially in the beginning. If you only acknowledge your living children you may feel a sense of betrayal, guilt, and even increased grief, but it may not be the appropriate time or situation to discuss it with strangers. They may not understand or feel comfortable having such a conversation. On the other hand, you may feel it important and necessary to count all your children in your response. No matter the response of others, you get to determine your own response.

There are a number of ways to handle this. You may have different answers for different situations and times. In a cashier's line with little time for discussion, you may say, "It's complicated," or "Too many," or "Not enough," and move on. Another way to handle it is to state a number and then change the subject or leave. Maybe on an airplane or on a subway you may be in a calmer and better space. You might say, "I

have two living children," or "I have two children who live with me and
two who live in my heart." Both invite conversation if others wish to
take it up. Perhaps you want no conversation about it at that moment, in
which case you might simply offer a number—including either all of
your children or just your living children—without further elaboration.

Prepare some answers that make you feel comfortable, loyal, and at
peace. Write them down, memorize them, and make them your own.
Once you have anticipated this question and how you can respond, it
may seem easier to go out in public knowing you are prepared.

> I could never—and still can't, eleven years down the track—answer
> this question without processing my answer. I don't think I ever will
> be able to. —Sarah

> I have my answers written on a recipe card in my purse. I practice
> them. Now I feel pretty comfortable that I have my options ready. I
> choose to not feel I am abandoning my babies who died. I do so
> much in my life to honor them [that] this is not even a worry I have.
> —Anonymous

> Raising two here on earth, and one who soars above. —Franchesca
> Cox, *Celebrating Pregnancy Again*

OVERPROTECTION

You have lost your innocence as a result of your loss. Since you know
that babies can die and that life is uncertain, it's hard to be nonchalant
when caring for your baby. You want to keep him safe. In fact, you may
be obsessed about it. Although obsession is not typical of most mothers,
the need to protect is. Accepting that your worldview has changed
forever can be a traumatic realization. How can parents of a child who
has died or who faces continual challenges trust this fragile world with
their living children?

Calling the nurse line or visiting the clinic often, having baby monitors placed in the baby's room, or simply not letting her out of your
sight may ease your mind. Sometimes overprotectiveness lasts for a
short while, but for some parents, it continues for many years. Being too
protective for too long can create a dependent child who lacks self-

confidence. Overprotectiveness can also result in a rebellious child who seeks thrills and dangerous activities. It is worthwhile to try and contain your overprotective impulses sooner rather than later. You may decide to allow yourself to feel what you feel—fear for their safety—on the inside but to show a more relaxed parenting style outwardly whenever you can.

> I would go outside his door and wait for him to wake up and cry. I'd have this horrible feeling he was dead inside, but I didn't want to let my irrational thoughts take over me. So I'd wait until I'd hear him cry. After a while, I started to trust life and stopped doing this, but it took almost a year. —Stephanie

> I am very protective of my little boy. He's three weeks old now and I just want to have him all to myself. I struggle when others, apart from my partner, want to feed him or change him. . . . It's as though I've got him and don't want to let him go! I hate playing "pass the parcel" with him at family events. I fear that every person who touches him is sick, and I don't want them near him. Are these normal feelings now that I have my little baby here in my arms after losing our first angel? Do any other moms feel the same? —A mom on Facebook

> I tried not to be overprotective, encouraging my sons to ski, jump on trampolines, ride snowmobiles, and even allowing them to ride on frozen lakes (one of my biggest stretches). Yet my oldest son described me as a WOPP (way overprotective parent). Now he runs with the bulls, ski dives, climbs mountains, and bungee jumps, to name a few. I fear he is either trying to give me a heart attack or getting back at me for those years of playing the protective game. Or maybe he just loves the adrenaline that comes with the thrills. In any case, I look back and wonder if I could have done things differently or if that is just his nature and I need to quell my fears. I pray a lot! —Anonymous

You need to be gentle with yourself and thoughtful of your child. Can you begin to trust again and take life one step at a time? You may want to find a subsequent pregnancy or birth support group or counselor to talk with as you work to stay healthy and to avoid becoming overprotective.

THE SAVIOR CHILD OR THE SPECIAL CHILD

This new baby will be a unique, special child to you. He may be so special that strangers can even tell that he is different in some way. Perhaps his birth healed you in a profound way. Or perhaps she awakened a gut-wrenching need in you to protect her from everything. Some parents adjust to having another baby quickly. They see a subsequent baby as they do their other living children. However, for some, the first subsequent child is forever unique. This child knows that she was born after a traumatic loss and is aware of the positive impact she has on her parents. This may even be discussed openly between family members.

Be honest and mindful about the situation. Don't put unrealistic expectations on your child, which could become unhelpful baggage for him. If need be, seek support as you adjust to parenting your special child.

> Phoenix was born on April 2, a miracle in my life. He picked me up when I thought my life would never truly be happy again. I look at him and I see happiness; I see hope, innocence, and pure love. I hold him and I am free; I smell him and I know all will be okay. He is the perfect baby, the perfect symbol of "recovery" for me, if there is such a thing. —Stephanie

WHAT TO TELL THE NEW CHILD?

How do you explain to your child that the baby who preceded her died? How do you explain the circumstances, or should you keep quiet? Although you don't have to tell other children anything if you don't want to, you also don't have to keep your loss a secret, either. It's up to you, but a common strategy is to tell young children early so that you won't have to have a big discussion someday. If it's right for you, keep saying your angel baby's name and telling stories. It will likely become natural within your family.

On the other hand, some parents prefer not to tell their children at a young age but to wait until they are older and can understand. You may find your children to be accepting and calm, easily riled up, or talkative about things that they don't understand or are upset about. Use your discretion; you know your children better than others.

One mother explains her experience telling her children:

> I told my kids, but not until they were in grade school. And frankly if
> I hadn't told them yet, I don't think it would have been a big deal.
> They weren't around, and he never lived. When I did tell them, they
> wouldn't stop bringing it up, which got annoying and weird. I don't
> regret telling them, but sometimes I wish I had waited until they
> were older. When someone asks me how many kids I have, I say four
> without hesitation, and sometimes *they* remind me—"No, you had
> five!" Sweet, yes, but sometimes I don't really feel like talking about
> it. Not because it hurts, even, but because it's over, and I'm good.
> Things worked out. Life has moved on and I'm at peace.

As your children ask questions or when you decide the time is right to
tell them, be sure to explain things in an age-appropriate way. Little
ones don't need—nor can they understand—long and complicated explanations. Start small then let the questions come. Chapter 20, "Supporting Your Children," offers many examples of how to have these
conversations with children of various ages. Even though it is primarily
about telling your living children about the recent death of a sibling, the
information will apply.

As a rule, children are resilient and accepting. Allow yourself to
grieve for her sibling in normal ways and to occasionally explain what
you are feeling and why. She will likely adjust well after you model that
you have. Honesty is usually the best policy. Try to make things simple
for her and to be genuine. At times, this will be sad; at other times, it
will be joyful. When you have birthday celebrations for your angel baby
with your subsequent children, you may notice a connectedness that
grows over time.

> I can tease my baby brother [who would have been eight] that way.
> After all, if he were alive, he would be teasing me. —Kellan, age
> seven

While you navigate parenthood of your subsequent baby, show your
love for each of your children and model openness and honesty about
your feelings and needs. You can include children who have died in
your daily lives and on holidays if you wish. In order to remember your
baby who died, your living children could buy toys for a child the age of
your baby and donate them to a local charity. There are many ways to

keep your children involved with and showing love for a sibling they never met.

You will find some excellent books on subsequent pregnancies that can help you. A few good ones are *Pregnancy after Loss*, by Joann O'Leary, *Trying Again: A Guide to Pregnancy after Miscarriage or Stillbirth*, by Ann Douglas, and *Celebrating Pregnancy Again*, by Franchesca Cox.

We hope that your rainbow baby will bring much sunshine into your life for many years to come.

TIPS AND ADVICE

- Write yourself a letter about your fears and anxiety but also about your joy, hope, and love toward this new baby. Remind yourself what made you decide to have another baby. Remind yourself that you will be a good parent.
- Become familiar with the common issues surrounding subsequent births after a loss. Know that you will feel anxious, scared, overprotective, and maybe even oversensitive. All of this is normal.
- Be aware of how you see and treat your new baby. Treating this child differently is common and normal, but be aware and mindful of how it may be positive or negative in the child's life or noticed by others in your life.
- Make sure the whole family communicates about issues that impact your parenting. Talk about issues as they arise.
- As suggested many times before, join a support group and hear advice from those who've gone on to have another baby. Talk to others who understand.
- Watch the movie *Return to Zero* (www.returntozerothemovie.com), the first Hollywood drama with stillbirth as its central theme. It is a poignant movie written and directed by Sean Hanish, who shares the heartbreaking true story of his stillborn and the difficult relationship between him and his wife as they live through the loss and embark on a subsequent pregnancy.

RESOURCES

During this difficult journey, it is important for you and your family to seek and receive the right kind of support. If your child is going to live with a disability, you will need many kinds of resources, including local support. If your baby died, you will need support at the time of loss, grief support, and connections to others who understand. If you have other children, are single, or are part of a couple, you will need guidance and help, so that you know that you are not alone.

One source of available support may be your hospital team. Ask the social worker, a hospice or bereavement counselor, or your midwife/obstetrician about referrals to someone who may be able to support you through this time. You may also seek support through support groups, resources, literature, friends and family, as well as relevant members of your community. You will find an extensive support system through social media on the Internet. Though do be careful. Some people and groups are not helpful and may even be hurtful, so be discriminating. If drama is common and the support you need is not evident, leave the group or site.

The following list of books, videos, websites, groups, and organizations may be useful to you as you travel the road of recovering from a prenatal diagnosis.

BOOKS

Prenatal Decision-making and Support

Difficult Decisions (Patricia Fertel and Joy Johnson)
Holding On & Letting Go (Vicki Culling)
Loving and Letting Go (Deborah L. Davis)
Precious Lives, Painful Choices: A Prenatal Decision-making Guide (Sherokee Ilse)
A Time to Decide, A Time to Heal (Molly Minnick)

Continuing the Pregnancy

Defiant Birth (Melinda Reist)
Family Lasts Forever: A Very Special Baby Book (a journal) (Sheila Frascht and Noel Andrews)
Giant Hero: One Couple's Journey through Loving and Letting Go of a Son with Potter's Syndrome (Tracey Ahrens)
A Gift of Time (Amy Kuebelbeck and Deborah L. Davis)
I Will Carry You (Angie Smith)
For the Love of Angela (Nancy Mayer-Whittington)
My Child, My Gift (Madeleine Nugent)
Not Compatible with Life: A Diary of Keeping Daniel (Kylie Sheffield)
Waiting with Gabriel (Amy Kuebelbeck)

Terminating the Pregnancy

Difficult Decisions (Centering Corporation)
Isaiah's Story (Jennifer Ross)
A Mother's Dilemma (Wendy Lyon)
Our Heartbreaking Choices: Forty-six Women Share Their Stories of Interrupting a Much-wanted Pregnancy (Christie Brooks)
Yesterday I Dreamed of Dreams (Molly Minnick)

Early Care and Memory-making

Empty Arms: Coping with Miscarriage, Stillbirth and Early Infant Death (Sherokee Ilse)
Love Lasts Forever: A Journal of Memories (Sheila Frascht and Noelle Andrews)
Meaningful Moments: Ritual and Reflection When a Child Dies (Rana Limbo and Kathy Kobler)
Mother Care: Physical Care and beyond after a Baby Dies (Sherokee Ilse, Inez Anderson, and Mary Funk)
When Hello Means Goodbye (Paul Kirk and Pat Schwiebert)

Saying Good-bye

Bittersweet . . . Hello Goodbye (National Share)
Caring for the Dead: Your Final Act of Love (Lisa Carlson)

Final Rights, Reclaiming the American Way of Death (Joshua Slocum and Lisa Carlson)
Planning a Precious Goodbye (Sherokee Ilse and Susan Erling Martinez)
When a Child Dies: A Resource for Families (Trina Charles)

Loss of a Baby Born as Part of a Multiple Pregnancy

Beginning with the End: A Memoir of Twin Loss and Healing (Mary Morgan)
The Diary (Lynne Schultz)
The Survivor (Lynne Schultz)
Twin Loss (Raymond Brandt)

For Fathers

A Bereaved Father (Steve Younis)
A Guide for Fathers (Tim Nelson)
Healing a Father's Grief (Compassionate Friends)
Men Don't Cry . . . Women Do (Terry L. Martin and Kenneth J. Doka)
Miscarriage: A Man's Book (Rick Wheat)
Strong and Tender: A Guide for the Father Whose Baby Dies (Pat Schwiebert)

For Couples

Couple Communication after a Baby Dies (Sherokee Ilse and Tim Nelson)
For Better or Worse: A Handbook for Couples Whose Child Has Died (Maribeth Doerr)
Grieving Parents: Surviving Loss as a Couple (Nathalie Himmelrich)
Healing Together: For Couples Grieving the Death of Their Baby (Marcie Lister and Sandra Lovell)
Men Are from Mars, Women Are from Venus (John Gray)
A Silent Sorrow: Pregnancy Loss: Guidance and Support for You and Your Family (Ingrid Kohn and Perry-Lynn Moffit)

For Singles or Teens

After the Loss of Your Baby: For Teen Mothers (Connie Nykiel)
Single Parent Grief (Sherokee Ilse)

Ongoing Parent Support

The Anguish of Loss (Julie Fritsch and Sherokee Ilse)
Baby Gone: True New Zealand Stories of Infertility, Miscarriage, Stillbirth, and Infant Loss (Jenny Douche)
Coping with the Holidays and Celebrations (Sherokee Ilse and Susan Erling)
Creative Acts of Healing after a Baby Dies (Judith van Praag)
Empty Cradle, Broken Heart (Deborah Davis)
From Crisis to Purpose: A Mother's Memoir (Tonya Dorsey)
Ghost Belly (Elizabeth Heineman)
Grief Unseen: Healing Pregnancy Loss through the Arts (Laura Seftel)
A Guide to Pregnancy after Miscarriage or Stillbirth (Ann Douglas)

Healing Your Heart after a Stillbirth (Alan Wofelt)
How to Survive the Loss of a Child (Catherine M. Sanders)
Life after Baby Loss (Nicola Miller-Clendon)
Life Touches Life: A Mother's Story of Stillbirth and Healing (Lorraine Ash)
Loss of a Baby, Death of a Dream (Margaret Nicol)
The Midwife and the Bereaved Family (Jane Warland)
Miscarriage: A Shattered Dream (Sherokee Ilse and Linda Hammer Burns)
Now That the Funeral Is Over: Understanding the Effects of Grief (Doris Zagdanski)
Only God Knows Why: A Mother's Memoir of Death and Rebirth (Amy Lyon)
Still Life with Baby (Elizabeth Heineman)
Sunshine after the Storm: A Survival Guide for the Grieving Mother (Alexa H. Bigwarfe,
    Regina Petsch, Amy Martin Hillis, Kathy Radign, Katia Bishop, et al.)
They Were Still Born: Personal Stories about Stillbirth (Janel Atlas)
Three Minus One: Stories of Parents' Love and Loss (Sean Hanish and Brooke Warner)
To Linger on Hot Coals: Collected Poetic Words from Grieving Women (Stephanie Cole and
    Catherine Bayly)
A Tribute to Tabitha-Rose: Stories of Baby & Infant Loss in New Zealand (Vicki Culling)

For Children

Always My Twin (Valerie Samuels)
Healthy Mindsets for Super Kids (Stephanie Azri)
I Wish I Could Hold Your Hand: A Child's Guide to Grief & Loss (Pat Palmer)
No New Baby (Marilyn Gryte)
Sibling Grief (Sherokee Ilse and Linda Hammer Burns)
Someone Came before You (Pat Schwiebert)
*Something Happened: A Book for Children and Parents Who Have Experienced Pregnancy
    Loss* (Cathy Blanford and Phyllis Childers)
Water Bugs and Dragonflies (Doris Stickney)
*We Were Going to Have a Baby, but We Had an Angel Instead: A Book about the Loss of a
    Brother or a Sister* (Pat Schwiebert)
What's Dead Mean? A Book to Help Children with Death (Doris Zagdanski)
Where Is Chloe? (Donna Wilkins and Nancy Munger)

Family Support

Grieving Grandparents (Sherokee Ilse and Lori Leininger)
What Family and Friends Can Do (Sherokee Ilse)

General Grief

*Coping with Grief and Loss: How to Recover from Loss and Overcome Feelings of Grief and
    Bereavement* (Anne C. Mapehrson)
Don't Take My Grief Away (Doug Manning)
The Grief Recovery Handbook (John W. James and Russell Friedman)
Remembering with Love: Messages of Hope for the First Year of Grieving and Beyond
    (Sherokee Ilse and Elizabeth Levang)
Tear Soup (Pat Schweibert and Chuck DeKlyen)
Understanding Mourning (Glen Davidson)
*Understanding Your Grief: Ten Essential Touchstones for Finding Hope and Healing Your
    Heart* (Alan D. Wolfelt)

When Bad Things Happen to Good People (Harold S. Kushner)

Subsequent Pregnancy

Another Baby? Maybe. 30 Questions on Pregnancy after Loss (Sherokee Ilse and Maribeth Doerr)
Celebrating Pregnancy Again: Restoring the Lost Joys of Pregnancy after the Loss of a Child (Franchesca Cox)
Journeys: Stories of Pregnancy after Loss (Amy Abbey)
Pregnancy after a Loss: A Guide to Pregnancy after a Miscarriage, Stillbirth, or Infant Death (Carol Cirulli Lanham)
Trying Again: A Guide to Pregnancy after Miscarriage, Stillbirth, and Infant Loss (Ann Douglas)
When Pregnancy Follows Loss (Joann O'Leary)

Special Needs Children

After the Tears: Parents Talk about Raising a Child with a Disability (Robin Simons)
The Boy in the Moon: A Father's Journey to Understand His Extraordinary Son (Ian Brown)
Breakthrough Parenting for Children with Special Needs: Raising the Bar of Expectations (Judy Winter)
Life Is a Gift and Other Lessons I'm Learning from My Daughters: A True Story (Jenny Miller)
My Baby Rides the Short Bus: The Unabashedly Human Experience of Raising Kids with Disabilities (Yantra Bertelli)
Special Children, Challenged Parents (Robert A. Naseef)

VIDEOS

Baby Darrius Noel's Home Memorial Service: www.youtube.com/watch?v=nCE45uqIHuA
Losing Layla (Vanessa Gorman): www.abc.net.au/tv/layla
Return To Zero (Sean Hanish): www.returntozerothemovie.com
What Family and Friends Can Do When a Baby Dies: http://wintergreenpress.org/shop/index.php?route=product/search&filter_name=shattered%20dreams

SUPPORT GROUPS AND WEBSITES

After a Prenatal Diagnosis—Neutral

Prenatal Diagnosis Support
PDS Australia is a support group for parents experiencing a pregnancy or infant loss following a poor prenatal diagnosis to families worldwide.
www.PDSAustralia.org

Baby Loss Family Advisors/Loss Doulas

Baby loss family advisors and loss doulas are certified, trained independent loss advisors who offer families guidance and companionship after the news of a loss or impending loss.
www.BabyLossFamilyAdvisors.org and www.LossDoulasInternational.com

Poor Prenatal Diagnosis (US)

This website offers informational services to parents worldwide after a poor prenatal diagnosis.

Antenatal Results Choices (UK)

ARC is a national charity that provides nondirective support and information to parents throughout the antenatal testing process.
www.arc-uk.org

For Those Who Continue the Pregnancy

Perinatal Hospice (US)

Perinatal Hospice and Palliative Care is for families who wish to continue their pregnancies with babies whose lives are expected to be brief.
http://perinatalhospice.org

Be Not Afraid

Be Not Afraid offers worldwide support to parents who have received poor or difficult prenatal diagnoses.
http://www.benotafraid.net/default.asp

Sufficient Grace Ministries

Sufficient Grace Ministries is a nonprofit, faith-based ministry that offers resources, trained volunteers for individual support, materials including mementos and literature, and connections to additional resources to families worldwide.
www.SufficientGraceMinistries.org

For Those Who End the Pregnancy

A Heartbreaking Choice

A Heartbreaking Choice is a worldwide support group that offers many services and emotional support for those parents who choose to interrupt their pregnancies after a poor prenatal diagnosis.
http://www.aheartbreakingchoice.com

A Loving Choice

A Loving Choice offers peer support through this online Facebook group. The group is closed and only parents who have terminated due to a fetal anomaly are allowed to join.
https://www.facebook.com/groups/8770390078

Rachel's Vineyard Ministry Healing

Rachel's Vineyard Ministry Healing is a biblically based retreat for all parents who seek healing after loss due to termination of a pregnancy.
www.rachelsvineyard.org

For Pregnancy and Infant Loss

SANDS (Australia, UK, and US)
SANDS promotes awareness, knowledge, support, and understanding following the death of a baby from the time of conception through to infancy.
www.sands.org.au
www.uk-sands.org
www.nationalshareoffice.com

Babies Remembered
Babies Remembered is a worldwide organization that supports families and caregivers by sharing extensive resources, organizations, literature, support options, awareness, educational opportunities, risk reduction and prevention, and legislative issues.
www.babiesremembered.org

The Compassionate Friends (Australia, UK, USA)
Compassionate Friends offers support, friendship, and understanding to parents who have had a child of any age die.
www.thecompassionatefriends.org.au
www.compassionatefriends.org
www.tcf.org.uk

Pregnancy Loss Australia
Pregnancy Loss Australia, formerly Teddy Love Club, is a national support program for bereaved families suffering from miscarriage, stillbirth, or termination for fetal abnormality and neonatal loss.
www.teddyloveclub.org.au

MISS Foundation (US)
The MISS Foundation is an international organization providing counseling, advocacy, research, and education services to families experiencing the death of a child.

Share (US)
Share Pregnancy and Infant Loss Support serves those touched by the tragic death of a baby through pregnancy loss, stillbirth, or during the first few months of life.
www.nationalshare.org

Star Legacy Foundation
The Star Legacy Foundation is a worldwide nonprofit organization dedicated to stillbirth research and education.
www.starlegacyfoundation.org

A Place to Remember
A Place to Remember is a worldwide organization that offers uplifting support resources for those who have been touched by a crisis in pregnancy or by the death of a baby. It offers the most comprehensive online store for baby loss materials including literature, videos, cards, gifts, and jewelry.
www.aplacetoremember.com

Centering Corporation
Centering Corporation is a worldwide organization that offers an extensive line of grief literature and provides caring workshops.
www.centering.org

OTHER SUPPORT RESOURCES

Memory Creation and Good-byes

The following websites offer memory-making items including jewelry, ornaments, photo montages, gowns, and so on.
www.APlacetoRemember.com
www.MyForeverChild.com
www.memory-of.com
www.myforeverprints.com
www.rememberingourbabies.net
www.castingkeepsakes.com
www.thecomfortcompany.net
www.aplacetoremember.com
www.griefwatch.com
www.alexandrasangelgifts.co.uk
www.tigerlilytrust.co.uk
www.borrowedmoments.co.uk
www.baby-burial-gowns.co.uk
www.keepituniquekeepsakes.com.au
www.theseashoreofremembrance.blogspot.com.au
www.littlesilverprints.com.au
www.memorialjewellery.com.au
www.portraitsbydana.com

Bringing Baby Home

Bring Your Baby Home

Bring Your Baby Home is a website for parents who are considering having time with their deceased baby at home. It provides information, stories, fact sheets, and support for bringing a baby home to say good-bye.
www.bringyourbabyhome.com

Cuddle Cots

Cuddle Cots are cooling systems that fit within a small cradle, cot, or bassinet that help make it possible for babies who have died to remain with their family members without having to be cooled in a morgue or mortuary. Many organizations and hospitals make them available to loan.
To buy worldwide:
http://flexmort.com/cuddle-cots
To buy in the United States:
www.storiesofbabiesbornstill.org
To borrow in Australia:
www.emerikuslandfoundation.org.au
http://pregnancylossaustralia.org.au
To borrow in the United Kingdom:
www.uk-sands.org
www.4louis.co.uk
To borrow in Canada:
http://tinyhandsofhope.ca
www.canuckplace.org

Subsequent Pregnancy

PALS

Pregnancy after Loss Support offers emotional and peer support to families who are trying to
   conceive following a pregnancy or infant loss. They also have a Facebook page.
www.pregnancyafterlosssupport.com

SPALS

SPALS is a warm and compassionate community of people who have experienced the loss of
   a child and share mutual support and information regarding subsequent pregnancies.
www.spals.com

Loss in Multiple Births

Center for Loss in Multiple Birth

Center for Loss in Multiple Birth offers services and support for families who have lost a
   baby who was born as part of a multiple birth.
www.climb-support.org

National Twin Loss Support

National Twin Loss Support provides support to parents who have lost a baby as part of a
   multiple birth, including but not limited to twins.
www.nationaltwinloss.org.au

OzMost

OzMost offers pregnancy loss support to families who have lost a baby as part of a multiple
   pregnancy. The support group is based in Australia, but it offers online peer support to
   families worldwide. The group is private so you will need to e-mail OzMOST@tpg.com.au
   in order to join.

SELECTED BIBLIOGRAPHY

Ahrens, Tracy. *Giant Hero*. New York: Infinity Publishing, 2008.

Azri, Stephanie. *Healthy Mindsets for Super Kids: A Resilience Programme for Children Aged 7–14*. London: Jessica Kingsley Publishers, 2013.

Azri, Stephanie. "Prenatal Diagnosis and Psychosocial Support." Thesis, Brisbane: Griffith University, 2014.

Brooks, Christie. *Our Heartbreaking Choices: Forty-six Women Share Their Stories of Interrupting a Much-wanted Pregnancy*. New York: iUniverse Publishing, 2008.

Charles, Trina, and Heidi Ciepielinski. *When a Child Dies: A Resource for Families*. Omaha, NE: Centering Corporation, 2005.

Cox, Franchesca. *Celebrating Pregnancy Again: Restoring the Lost Joys of Pregnancy after the Loss of a Child*. Create Space: Independent Publishing, 2013.

Culling, Vicki. *Holding On & Letting Go: Facing an Unexpected Diagnosis in Pregnancy*. Wellington, NZ: Vicki Culling Associates, 2013.

Doerr, Maribeth. *For Better, For More: For Couples Whose Child Has Died*. Omaha, NE: Centering Corporation, 1992.

Douglas, Ann. *A Guide to Pregnancy after Miscarriage or Stillbirth* Lanham, MD: Taylor Trade Publishing, 2000.

Gray, John. *Men Are from Mars, Women Are from Venus: A Practical Guide for Improving Communication and Getting What You Want in Your Relationships*. NY: HarperCollins, 1992.

Heineman, Elizabeth. *Still Life with Baby*. Millenium Writings, 2012.

Himmelrich, Nathalie. *Grieving Parents—Surviving Loss As a Couple*. Independent Publishing, 2014.

Ilse, Sherokee. *Empty Arms: Coping with Miscarriage, Stillbirth and Infant Death*. Wayzata, MN: Wintergreen Press, 2013.

Ilse, Sherokee. *Single Parent Grief*. Place to Remember, 2007.

Ilse, Sherokee. *Precious Lives, Painful Choices: A Prenatal Decision-making Guide*. Wayzata MN: Wintergreen Press, 1993.

Ilse, Sherokee, and Maribeth Doerr. *Another Baby? Maybe. 30 Questions on Pregnancy after Loss*. Wayzata, MN: Wintergreen Press, 2009.

Ilse, Sherokee, Inez Anderson, and Mary Funk,. *Mother Care: Physical Care and beyond after a Baby Dies*. Wayzata, MN: Wintergreen Press, 2002.

Ilse, Sherokee, and Susan Erling. *Coping with the Holidays and Celebrations*. St. Paul, MN: A Place to Remember.

Ilse, Sherokee, and Susan Erling Martinez. *Planning a Precious Goodbye*. Wayzata, MN: Wintergreen Press, 2013.

Ilse, Sherokee, and Tim Nelson. *Couple Communication after a Baby Dies: Differing Perspectives*. Place to Remember, 2009.

Klaus, M., and J. H. Kennell, *Parent-to-infant Attachment*. St. Louis: Mosby, 1976.

Kuebelbeck, Amy. *Waiting with Gabriel: A Story of Cherishing a Baby's Brief Life*. Chicago: Loyola Press, 2003.

Kuebelbeck, Amy, and Deborah L. Davis. *A Gift of Time: Continuing Your Pregnancy When Your Baby's Life Is Expected to Be Brief*. Baltimore: Johns Hopkins University Press, 2011.

Lanham, Carol Cirulli. *Pregnancy after a Loss: A Guide to Pregnancy after a Miscarriage, Stillbirth, or Infant Death*. New York: Berkley Books, 1999.

O'Leary, Joann. *Pregnancy after Loss*. Minneapolis, MN: Lambert Academic Publishing, 2010.

Ross, Jennifer. *Isaiah's Story*. Greenville, SC: Ambassador International, 2014.

Schwiebert, Pat, and Paul Kirk. *When Hello Means Goodbye: A Guide for Parents Whose Child Dies before Birth, at Birth or Shortly after Birth*. Portland, OR: Perinatal Loss, 2012.

ABOUT THE AUTHORS

Stephanie Azri has worked as a child and family clinical social worker with a major in women's health. Her area of expertise has been in supporting women around pregnancy and family issues. In 2002, Stephanie, pregnant with her third child, received an adverse prenatal diagnosis that changed her life in many ways. She faced the heartbreaking decision of having to decide her pregnancy outcome. She realized that no matter what she chose, she would be changed forever and found that scarce support was available to women and their families going through this traumatic journey.

Stephanie has written multiple academic journal articles, magazine articles, blog posts, and books that are available worldwide. She also presents regularly at conferences about women's health issues.

Her PhD, undertaken through the school of human services and social work from Griffith University, Australia, focuses on the impact of psychosocial support on women's well-being after adverse prenatal diagnoses. Her findings highlighted that women were concerned about some aspects of their care after a poor prenatal diagnosis and were keen to advocate for wider and specific support. Stephanie presented the Skills, Assessment, Referral and Follow up (SARF) model as a proposed method of providing adequate care to women in the health system, and this model is currently being further investigated in clinical settings.

She is the founder and coordinator of PDS Australia (Prenatal Diagnosis Support Australia), a support group for women who have received adverse prenatal diagnoses. The support group offers e-mail support, discussion forums, peer support, referrals to services, and advocacy. It also holds a strong research agenda with academic and clinical input from various experts in the field.

Sherokee Ilse is an author, parent advocate, international speaker, and trainer in the infant loss world since months after her son Brennan was stillborn at term. She had an earlier miscarriage (Marama) and later an ectopic pregnancy (Bryna), along with two wonderful, living sons. She has dedicated her life to helping other bereaved parents.

She is the author of *Empty Arms: Coping with Miscarriage, Stillbirth, and Infant Death*, one of the first self-help books for newly bereaved parents. During the past thirty years she has written or cowritten seventeen more books and booklets for families and their caregivers on the subject of perinatal baby loss.

Cofounder of a national nonprofit pregnancy and infant loss organization, she co-led the initiative to make October Pregnancy and Infant Loss Awareness Month and has spoken at thousands of conferences, workshops, in-services, and support groups. Sherokee is president of company Wintergreen Press and Babies Remembered, and she cofounded a certification program for Baby Loss Doulas, also called Baby Loss Family Advisors. This new paradigm of well-trained loss doulas/advisors helps bereaved families make plans for their baby's birth (including miscarriage and stillbirth as well as other types of early losses), supports them while in the hospital, and helps them transition to home. www.BabyLossFamilyAdvisors.org

Sherokee has specifically worked to support families who have a poor prenatal outcome diagnosis. Her book, *Precious Lives, Painful Choices: A Prenatal Decision-making Guide*, is shared by genetic counselors and other caregivers with parents as soon as they learn the bad news and are asked to make heartbreaking decisions.